Dx/Rx:

Genitourinary Oncology
Cancer of the Kidneys, Bladder, and Testis
Second Edition

Matthew D. Galsky, MD
Mount Sinai School of Medicine
Director, Genitourinary Medical Oncology
The Tisch Cancer Institute
New York, New York

Series Editor: Manish A. Shah, MD
Memorial Sloan-Kettering Cancer Center
Department of Medicine
GI Oncology Service
New York, New York

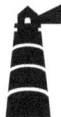

JONES & BARTLETT
L E A R N I N G

World Headquarters
Jones & Bartlett Learning
40 Tall Pine Drive
Sudbury, MA 01776
978-443-5000
info@jblearning.com
www.jblearning.com

Jones & Bartlett Learning Canada
6339 Ormindale Way
Mississauga, Ontario L5V 1J2
Canada

Jones & Bartlett Learning International
Barb House, Barb Mews
London W6 7PA
United Kingdom

Jones & Bartlett Learning books and products are available through most bookstores and
online booksellers. To contact Jones & Bartlett Learning directly, call 800-832-0034,
fax 978-443-8000, or visit our website, www.jblearning.com.

Substantial discounts on bulk quantities of Jones & Bartlett Learning publications are
available to corporations, professional associations, and other qualified organizations.
For details and specific discount information, contact the special sales department
at Jones & Bartlett Learning via the above contact information or send an email to
specialsales@jblearning.com.

The author, editor, and publisher have made every effort to provide accurate information.
However, they are not responsible for errors, omissions, or for any outcomes related to the
use of the contents of this book and take no responsibility for the use of the products
and procedures described. Treatments and side effects described in this book may not be
applicable to all people; likewise, some people may require a dose or experience a side
effect that is not described herein. Drugs and medical devices are discussed that may have
limited availability controlled by the Food and Drug Administration (FDA) for use only in a
research study or clinical trial. Research, clinical practice, and government regulations often
change the accepted standard in this field. When consideration is being given to use of any
drug in the clinical setting, the healthcare provider or reader is responsible for determining
FDA status of the drug, reading the package insert, and reviewing prescribing information
for the most up-to-date recommendations on dose, precautions, and contraindications, and
determining the appropriate usage for the product. This is especially important in the case
of drugs that are new or seldom used.

Production Credits

Executive Publisher: Christopher Davis
Associate Editor: Laura Burns
Associate Production Editor: Jill Morton
Marketing Manager: Rebecca Rockel
V.P., Manufacturing and Inventory Control:
 Therese Connell
Composition: Circle Graphics, Inc.
Cover Design: Kate Ternullo
Cover Image: © Sebastian Kaulitzki/
 ShutterStock, Inc.
Printing and Binding: Malloy Incorporated
Cover Printing: Malloy Incorporated

Library of Congress Cataloging-in-Publication Data
Galsky, Matthew D.
 Dx/Rx. Genitourinary oncology : cancer of the kidneys, bladder, and testis / by Matthew D.
Galsky. — 2nd ed.
 p. ; cm.
 Genitourinary oncology
 Includes bibliographical references and index.
 ISBN-13: 978-0-7637-9298-5
 ISBN-10: 0-7637-9298-5
 1. Kidneys—Cancer—Handbooks, manuals, etc. 2. Bladder—Cancer—Handbooks, manuals,
etc. 3. Testis—Cancer—Handbooks, manuals, etc. I. Title. II. Title: Genitourinary oncology.
 [DNLM: 1. Kidney Neoplasms—diagnosis—Handbooks. 2. Kidney Neoplasms—therapy—
Handbooks. 3. Testicular Neoplasms—diagnosis—Handbooks. 4. Testicular Neoplasms—
therapy—Handbooks. 5. Urinary Bladder Neoplasms—diagnosis—Handbooks. 6. Urinary
Bladder Neoplasms—therapy—Handbooks. WJ 39]
 RC280.K5G35 2012
 616.99'461—dc22
                                        2011004739
6048

Printed in the United States of America
15 14 13 12 11   10 9 8 7 6 5 4 3 2 1

Dedication

This book is dedicated to all of the patients who have entrusted me with their care over the years. I have learned countless lessons from each and every one of them.

Contents

Editor's Preface

I would like to welcome you to this second edition of *Dx/Rx: Genitourinary Oncology* by Matthew D. Galsky, MD. This book focuses on the diagnosis and management of nonprostate genitourinary malignancies, including bladder cancer, renal cell carcinoma, and germ cell malignancies. These cancers have seen significant progress over the past few years, including the ongoing development and approval of new, targeted therapies including everolimus and bevacizumab for renal cell carcinoma. The book is formatted in easy-to-read bulleted text and tables and is divided into chapters that quite expertly separate these malignancies so as to provide easy access for reference to the diagnosis and management of these complex diseases. I am certain that you will find this book, as well as all of the books in the Dx/Rx Oncology Series, an integral part of your reference arsenal in the management of these common and changing cancers of the genitourinary tract.

Manish A. Shah, MD

Acknowledgments

I would like to thank my wife and children for allowing me the time to complete this book.

Introduction

Genitourinary oncology is a diverse and fascinating field. The three malignancies covered in this book, testicular cancer, bladder cancer, and kidney cancer, are certainly a testament to this fact. Testicular cancer represents one of the major success stories in solid tumor oncology. A disease that once commonly caused the death of afflicted young men is now routinely cured due to multidisciplinary efforts over the past several decades. Bladder cancer is a prime example of the promise and pitfalls of combination chemotherapy, a disease highlighted by extreme chemosensitivity, but rare durable responses in the metastatic setting. Kidney cancer embodies the future of oncology, with recent effective treatments developed based on uncovering the molecular mechanisms driving this disease. My hope is that this book will provide a practical reference for the routine management of these diseases.

Cancers of the Bladder/Urothelial Tract

CHAPTER 1

Bladder Cancer: Epidemiology and Risk Factors

■ Epidemiology

- Cancer of the urinary bladder ranks eleventh in incidence among cancers worldwide.
- Internationally, approximately 310,000 new cases are diagnosed each year.
- In the United States, cancer of the urinary bladder is the fourth most common cancer in men and the tenth most common cancer in women.
- Approximately 60,000 individuals are diagnosed with bladder cancer, and approximately 13,000 individuals will die from this disease each year in the United States.[1]
- The majority of patients (approximately 75%) present with localized disease.

■ Demographics

- The incidence of bladder cancer increases with age.
- Approximately 80% of patients are diagnosed after the age of 60.
- Bladder cancer is more common in men than in women (with a ratio of 2:1 to 4:1).

■ Risk Factors

- Several chemical and environmental exposures have been linked to the development of bladder cancer. However, in many cases, the long latency period between the exposure and development of clinical disease has limited the ability to establish causality.

- Tobacco smoking
  - Cigarette smoking is the most important risk factor for bladder cancer and is thought to contribute to one or two of every three cases of bladder cancer diagnosed.[2]
- Industry-related carcinogens
  - Multiple compounds have been implicated. The majority of these carcinogens are aromatic amines.
  - Occupations linked to the development of bladder cancer include the aluminum, dye, paint, petroleum, rubber, and textile industries. Occupations involving exposure to "combustion gases," including chimney sweeps, truck drivers, and garage or gas station workers, have also been associated with an increased risk.[3]
- Diet
  - Consumption of fried or fatty foods may increase the risk of developing bladder cancer.[4]
  - The quality of drinking water, through the by-products of water chlorination and the concentration of arsenic, has also been associated with an increased risk.[5]
- Drugs
  - Phenacetin (an analgesic agent) has been associated with chronic renal disease and development of cancers of the bladder, ureter, and renal pelvis.[6]
  - Cyclophosphamide (an immunosuppressant/cytotoxic agent) increases the risk of bladder cancer up to ninefold with a latency period of generally less than 10 years.[7]
- Infectious agents
  - Schistosomiasis, caused by the trematode *Schistosoma haematobium*, is endemic to the Middle East, Southeast Asia, and Africa. Bilharzial bladder disease, secondary to infection with *S. haematobium*, has been linked to the development of carcinoma of the bladder. The majority of these cases are squamous cell carcinomas, as opposed to the vast majority of bladder cancer cases in the United States, which are transitional cell carcinomas.[8]

■ References

1. Jemal A, Siegel R, Ward E, et al. Cancer statistics, 2007. *CA Cancer J Clin.* 2007;57:43–66.
2. Burch JD, Rohan TE, Howe GR, et al. Risk of bladder cancer by source and type of tobacco exposure: a case-control study. *Int J Cancer.* 1989;44:622–628.
3. Silverman DT, Hartge P, Morrison AS, et al. Epidemiology of bladder cancer. *Hematol Oncol Clin North Am.* 1992; 6:1–30.
4. Steineck G, Hagman U, Gerhardsson M, et al. Vitamin A supplements, fried foods, fat and urothelial cancer. A case-referent study in Stockholm in 1985–87. *Int J Cancer.* 1990;45:1006–1011.
5. Cantor KP, Lynch CF, Hildesheim ME, et al. Drinking water source and chlorination byproducts. I. Risk of bladder cancer. *Epidemiology.* 1998;9:21–28.
6. Burkart TE. Bladder carcinoma and phenacetin. *Ann Intern Med.* 1980;92:131.
7. O'Keane JC. Carcinoma of the urinary bladder after treatment with cyclophosphamide. *N Engl J Med.* 1988;319:871.
8. Ross AG, Bartley PB, Sleigh AC, et al. Schistosomiasis. *N Engl J Med.* 2002;346:1212–1220.

Bladder Cancer: Diagnosis, Pathology, and Staging

■ Symptoms

- Hematuria is the most common presenting symptom of bladder cancer. The hematuria is typically gross, painless, and intermittent.
  - Asymptomatic microscopic hematuria is rarely due to bladder cancer. In a population-based study, 13% of individuals had microscopic hematuria but only 0.4% were diagnosed with bladder cancer.[1]
- Pain is typically related to locally advanced or metastatic disease.
- Irritative voiding symptoms can occur (e.g., dysuria, frequency, urgency).
- Constitutional symptoms are typically an indication of advanced disease (e.g., fatigue, weight loss, anorexia).

■ Initial Diagnostic Workup

- Gross hematuria in an individual >40 years old is urothelial carcinoma until proven otherwise (provided there is no evidence of glomerular bleeding).
- Gross hematuria, or other signs or symptoms suggestive of urothelial carcinoma, warrants the following evaluation:
  - Urine cytology
    - Greatest sensitivity (approximately 90%) for detection of carcinoma in situ.
  - Cystoscopy
    - Mainstay of diagnosis and evaluation of bladder cancer.
    - Allows direct visualization of the urethra and inner walls of the bladder and allows biopsies of suspicious sites.

- Upper urinary tract evaluation
  - Evaluation of the upper urinary tract is essential because urothelial carcinomas may be located at any site from the renal pelvis to the urethra and may be multifocal. This also allows visualization of the renal parenchyma to rule out a renal cell carcinoma:
    - Computed tomography (CT) scan of the abdomen and pelvis with urography, or
    - Intravenous pyelography plus renal ultrasound
- Novel urine-based assays have been developed to enhance the detection of bladder cancer. Their role in the initial diagnosis of bladder cancer is in evolution.
  - NMP 22: A point-of-care, urine-based assay to detect nuclear matrix protein 22 is approved for the diagnosis of bladder cancer. This assay was evaluated in a prospective study of 1,331 individuals with risk factors for bladder cancer.[2] The sensitivity and specificity of the NMP 22 assay were 55% and 85%, respectively, compared with the sensitivity and specificity of cytology, which were 15% and 99%, respectively.
- Ultimately, the diagnosis of urothelial carcinoma is made upon review of a biopsy of an abnormal site within the urothelial tract by a pathologist.

■ Pathology

- The lining of the urinary tract, the urothelium, extends from the renal pelvis to the urethra. The term *urothelial carcinoma* is used for cancers that arise at any site within the urothelial tract.
- The majority of cancers of the urothelial tract are transitional cell carcinomas (90–95% of cases in the United States).
- Approximately 90% of urothelial carcinomas develop within the bladder, whereas 8% develop in the renal pelvis and 2% develop in the ureters or urethra.
- Many patients develop multifocal urothelial tumors, presenting either synchronously or metachronously. Two main mechanisms have been proposed to account for the multifocal nature of urothelial carcinomas, and

both are likely involved. The "field cancerization effect" suggests that multifocal tumors develop because the entire urothelial tract is exposed to the same carcinogens. Alternatively, genetic studies have demonstrated that the majority of multifocal sites of urothelial carcinoma are monoclonal, and seeding of malignant cells throughout the urothelial tract may be responsible.

- Less common histologies:[3]
  - Squamous cell carcinoma
    - Rare in the United States; however, in *Schistosoma haematobium*–endemic regions, squamous cell carcinomas predominate.
  - Adenocarcinoma
    - May develop in the remnant of the urachus (urachal adenocarcinoma) or at other sites within the bladder.
  - Small cell carcinoma
  - Nonepithelial subtypes (e.g., sarcomas, melanomas) are extremely rare.
- Tumor grade
  - Urothelial carcinomas are classified as low grade or high grade based on their resemblance to normal urothelial tissue.
  - The majority of invasive bladder cancers are high grade; superficial bladder cancers may be low grade or high grade.

■ Staging of Bladder Cancer

- The goal of bladder cancer staging is to determine the local extent of the tumor in the bladder (and to determine if the cancer is resectable), whether there are regional lymph nodes involved with cancer, and whether there are distant metastases present.
- The following examinations are utilized to stage bladder cancer and constitute clinical staging:
  - Cystoscopy/transurethral resection of bladder tumor (TURBT)
    - Visible lesions in the bladder are resected (TURBT) to determine the histologic type of bladder cancer

and the depth of invasion into the bladder wall (the T stage).

- If urine cytology reveals malignant cells but cystoscopy reveals no evidence of tumor in the bladder or urethra, evaluation of the upper urinary tracts (ureters and renal pelvis) is essential.

- Exam under anesthesia
  - A bimanual exam is performed at the time of cystoscopy to determine the presence of a palpable mass. If a mass is present, the mobility of the mass is then noted.
  - If a mass is palpated, the examination is repeated after TURBT to determine if the mass is still palpable. This allows the differentiation of clinical stage T2 and clinical stage T3 disease.
  - If the mass is not mobile (a "fixed" mass), this represents clinical stage T4b disease, which by definition is an unresectable tumor.

- CT scans
  - CT scans are often utilized for evaluating the local extent of tumor, lymph node involvement, and the presence of distant metastases.
  - The sensitivity and specificity of CT scans for regional lymph node involvement are low, and biopsies of suspicious lymph nodes should be performed for confirmation if this will result in a change in management.

- Bone scans
  - Bone scans are considered for patients with symptoms worrisome for bone metastases or for patients with elevations in the serum alkaline phosphatase level.

- Bladder cancers are staged using the TNM (tumor, node, metastasis) staging system.
  - *Clinical staging* includes information derived from the cystoscopy, exam under anesthesia (EUA), TURBT, and radiographic imaging.
  - *Pathologic staging* includes information derived from review of the entire bladder specimen after cystectomy.

- An understanding of bladder wall anatomy is necessary to understand the T-stage categorization scheme. The wall of the bladder consists of four layers:
  - *Urothelium*: The innermost epithelial lining of the bladder.
  - *Lamina propria*: Separated from the urothelium by the basement membrane.
  - *Muscularis propria*: Thick layer of muscle (detrusor muscle) surrounding the lamina propria.
  - *Serosa*: The outermost layer of the bladder.
- TNM staging (see **Tables 2.1** and **2.2** for stage groupings).

Table 2.1   TNM Staging in Bladder Cancer

T Stage (Primary Tumor)	
Tis	Carcinoma in situ: "flat tumor"
Ta	Noninvasive papillary carcinoma
T1	Tumor invades subepithelial connective tissue
T2	Tumor invades muscularis propria
	T2a—tumor invades superficial muscularis propria (inner half)
	T2b—tumor invades deep muscularis propria (outer half)
T3	Tumor invades perivesical tissue
	T3a—microscopically
	T3b—macroscopically (extravesical mass)
T4	Tumor invades any of the following: prostatic stroma, seminal vesicles, uterus, vagina, pelvic wall, abdominal wall
	T4a—tumor invades prostatic stroma, uterus, or vagina
	T4b—tumor invades pelvic wall, abdominal wall

(Continues)

Table 2.1 TNM Staging in Bladder Cancer (Continued)

N Stage (Lymph Nodes)	
N0	No regional lymph node metastases
N1	Single regional lymph node metastasis in the true pelvis (hypogastric, obturator, external iliac, or presacral lymph node)
N2	Multiple regional lymph node metastasis in the true pelvis (hypogastric, obturator, external iliac, or presacral lymph node metastasis)
N3	Lymph node metastasis to the colon iliac lymph nodes
M Stage (Metastases)	
M0	No distant metastasis
M1	Distant metastasis

Source: Used with the permission of the American Joint Committee on Cancer (AJCC), Chicago, Illinois. The original source for this material is the *AJCC Cancer Staging Manual,* Seventh Edition (2010), published by Springer Science and Business Media LLC, www.springer.com.

Table 2.2 Bladder Cancer Stage Groupings

Stage Grouping	T Stage	N Stage	M Stage
0a	Ta	N0	M0
0is	Tis	N0	M0
I	T1	N0	M0
II	T2a	N0	M0
	T2b	N0	M0
III	T3a	N0	M0
	T3b	N0	M0
IV	T4a	N0	M0
	T4b	N0	M0
	Any T	N1-3	M0
	Any T	Any N	M1

Source: Used with the permission of the American Joint Committee on Cancer (AJCC), Chicago, Illinois. The original source for this material is the *AJCC Cancer Staging Manual,* Seventh Edition (2010), published by Springer Science and Business Media LLC, www.springer.com.

■ References

1. Mohr DN, Offord KP, Owen RA, et al. Asymptomatic micro-hematuria and urologic disease. A population-based study. *JAMA.* 1986;256:224–229.
2. Grossman HB, Messing E, Soloway M, et al. Detection of bladder cancer using a point-of-care proteomic assay. *JAMA.* 2005;293:810–816.
3. Manunta A, Vincendeau S, Kiriakou G, et al. Non-transitional cell bladder carcinomas. *BJU Int.* 2005;95:497–502.

CHAPTER 3

Superficial Bladder Cancer

■ Definition

▪ Superficial bladder cancer includes the following T stages:
  ● Tis: Carcinoma in situ.
  ● Ta: Papillary tumor located above the basement membrane.
  ● T1: Tumor extending into the lamina propria but not the muscularis propria.
▪ Given their disparate natural histories, some experts have proposed that the term *superficial bladder cancer* be restricted to patients with Ta tumors and the term *noninvasive bladder cancer* be used to refer to the more aggressive Tis and T1 tumors.[1]

■ Public Health Implications

▪ Bladder cancer is the fourth most common cancer in men and the eighth most common cancer in women worldwide.
▪ Of the approximately 60,000 new cases of bladder cancer per year in the United States, 70–80% are superficial bladder cancers.
▪ Given the need for frequent cystoscopies, transurethral resections, and intravesical therapy, superficial bladder cancer is a significant economic burden. The estimated lifetime cost of treating a patient presenting with superficial disease is $65,000.[2]

■ Prognosis

▪ Prognostic factors in superficial bladder cancer are critical in identifying not only patients at risk for recurrence but also, more importantly, those patients at risk for progression (development of more invasive tumors). The latter group of patients will ultimately be at risk for bladder cancer–associated mortality.

- T stage and grade
  - Low-grade papillary tumors (Ta) frequently recur after resection but rarely progress to more invasive tumors (≈4% rate of progression in one series). High-grade papillary tumors are associated with a higher rate of progression to more invasive tumors (≈23% in one series).[3]
  - Carcinoma in situ is generally high grade at presentation and associated with a high rate of progression to more invasive tumors.[4]
  - The vast majority of T1 tumors are high grade at presentation. Approximately 50% of patients with T1 tumors will develop muscle-invasive disease within 10 years.[5] The 5-year mortality rate of high-grade pathologic stage T1 tumors is as high as 24%.[6]
- Number of tumors at presentation
  - Patients with solitary superficial tumors are less likely to develop recurrence than patients with multiple superficial tumors at the time of presentation.[7]
- Size of tumors
  - Tumor sizes greater than 3–5 cm have been correlated with worse outcomes.[8]
- Number and frequency of recurrences
  - The interval between tumor recurrences is associated with the likelihood of subsequent recurrences.[9]
  - The risk of progression to more invasive tumors has not been definitively associated with the number of superficial recurrences.[10]

■ Treatment of Superficial Bladder Cancer

- *Treatment based on risk stratification*: Based on the known prognostic factors, patients with superficial bladder cancer are often divided into two groups based on their risk for progression and bladder cancer–associated mortality (see **Table 3.1**):
  - *Low risk*: Generally managed by TURBT (complete transurethral resection of all visible bladder tumor through the cystoscope) alone followed by surveillance

Table 3.1   Risk Stratification in Superficial Bladder Cancer

Low Risk	High Risk
Low grade	High grade
Ta tumors	T1 tumors
<3 cm	≥3 cm
≤3 lesions	>3 lesions
Long interval between recurrences	Short interval between recurrences
	Diffuse carcinoma in situ

- *High risk*: Generally managed by TURBT plus intra-vesical therapy followed by surveillance
- *High-grade T1 disease:* High-grade T1 disease is the most aggressive of the superficial bladder lesions. There is much controversy about the optimal management of these tumors. A standard approach is a complete TURBT followed by adjuvant intravesical bacillus Calmette-Guérin (BCG). Despite this approach, data suggest that approximately one-third of patients will survive with their bladder intact, another one-third will survive but ultimately require cystectomy, and one-third will succumb to progressive urothelial carcinoma.[5] As a result, some experts advocate early cystectomy for patients with high-grade T1 disease. A randomized trial of adjuvant radiation therapy after complete resection of high-grade T1 disease did not demonstrate a delay in progression or death with the addition of radiation therapy.[11]
- *Carcinoma in situ:* Carcinoma in situ is treated with intravesical instillation of BCG followed by surveillance (see below).
- Intravesical therapy
  - Instillation of chemotherapy or other therapeutic agent directly into the bladder with the goal of eradicating residual cancer cells to reduce the risk of recurrence and progression after TURBT.

- Bacillus Calmette-Guérin (BCG)
  - Mechanism
    - Live attenuated strain of *Mycobacterium bovis.*
    - The most commonly used and most efficacious agent for intravesical therapy.
    - The precise mechanism of antitumor activity is unclear, although it is linked to stimulation of local immune response.
  - Administration
    - Typically instilled into the bladder weekly for 6 weeks.
    - Retained in the bladder for 2 hours at each treatment.
    - Maintenance intravesical BCG after a 6-week induction course is controversial. A randomized trial demonstrated an improvement in disease-free survival but not in overall survival.[12]
  - Efficacy
    - Intravesical BCG after TURBT for high-risk superficial bladder cancer is associated with a decreased risk of progression and a decreased need for subsequent cystectomy.[13] The impact of BCG on survival is controversial, although some studies have demonstrated a decrease in bladder cancer–associated mortality.[14]
    - Intravesical BCG is the treatment of choice for carcinoma in situ. Treatment is associated with a complete response rate of 60% and a median duration of response of over 3 years.[15]
    - Several other intravesical agents (including mitomycin, doxorubicin, and epirubicin) have been compared with BCG in randomized trials; none has proven superior.[16–19]
  - Adverse events
    - Irritative bladder symptoms (urinary frequency, dysuria).
    - Local and systemic infectious complications rarely occur after BCG administration. The risk of sepsis is estimated at 1 in 15,000 patients.[20]
- *Intravesical chemotherapy*: Other intravesical agents have shown activity in patients as initial therapy for

superficial bladder cancer and as treatment for patients who have persistent/recurrent disease following BCG. The anthracyclines and mitomycin reduce the risk of early recurrence (recurrence within 1 year) from low-grade Ta tumors by 33–50%. None of these agents has been proven to improve survival or risk of progression.[21]

- Mitomycin
- Anthracyclines (doxorubicin, epirubicin, valrubicin)
- Gemcitabine
- Docetaxel

■ Surveillance After Treatment of Superficial Bladder Cancer

- Surveillance after initial treatment for superficial bladder cancer is critical for early detection of recurrent/progressive tumors.
- Surveillance recommendations vary somewhat based on the source of the recommendations. A common surveillance approach is as follows:
  - Repeat cystoscopy and urine cytology every 3 months for 2 years, followed by every 6 months for 2 years, followed by annually (in the absence of recurrence).
  - Evaluation of the upper urinary tracts should be performed every 1–2 years to evaluate for metachronous lesions.
- Less frequent surveillance may be appropriate for patients with low-grade pTa tumors with no evidence of recurrence on initial posttreatment cystoscopy.
- Adherence with surveillance strategies in practice likely differs substantially from standard recommendations. In an analysis of Surveillance Epidemiology and End Results (SEER) program Medicare-linked data, only 40% of patients completed all of the recommended cystoscopies during the follow-up period.[22]
- *Urine biomarkers:* The benefit of several urine biomarkers (e.g., NMP 22 test) in surveillance for recurrence after treatment of superficial bladder cancer has been evaluated in clinical trials. The role of these biomarkers when added to standard surveillance strategies is in evolution.

■ References

1. Abel PD, Hall RR, Williams G. Should pT1 transitional cell cancers of the bladder still be classified as superficial? *Br J Urol.* 1988;62:235–239.
2. Avritscher EB, Cooksley CD, Grossman HB, et al. Clinical model of lifetime cost of treating bladder cancer and associated complications. *Urology.* 2006;68:549–553.
3. Holmang S, Andius P, Hedelin H, et al. Stage progression in Ta papillary urothelial tumors: relationship to grade, immunohistochemical expression of tumor markers, mitotic frequency and DNA ploidy. *J Urol.* 2001;165:1124–1128; discussion 1128–1130.
4. Lamm DL. Carcinoma in situ. *Urol Clin North Am.* 1992; 19:499–508.
5. Shahin O, Thalmann GN, Rentsch C, et al. A retrospective analysis of 153 patients treated with or without intravesical bacillus Calmette-Guerin for primary stage T1 grade 3 bladder cancer: recurrence, progression and survival. *J Urol.* 2003;169:96–100; discussion 100.
6. Anderstrom C, Johansson S, Nilsson S. The significance of lamina propria invasion on the prognosis of patients with bladder tumors. *J Urol.* 1980;124:23–26.
7. Dalesio O, Schulman CC, Sylvester R, et al. Prognostic factors in superficial bladder tumors. A study of the European Organization for Research on Treatment of Cancer: Genitourinary Tract Cancer Cooperative Group. *J Urol.* 1983;129:730–733.
8. Kurth KH, Denis L, Bouffioux C, et al. Factors affecting recurrence and progression in superficial bladder tumours. *Eur J Cancer.* 1995;31A:1840–1846.
9. Fitzpatrick JM, West AB, Butler MR, et al. Superficial bladder tumors (stage pTa, grades 1 and 2): the importance of recurrence pattern following initial resection. *J Urol.* 1986;135:920–922.
10. Torti FM, Lum BL, Aston D, et al. Superficial bladder cancer: the primacy of grade in the development of invasive disease. *J Clin Oncol.* 1987;5:125–130.
11. Harland SJ, United Kingdom National Cancer Research Institute Bladder Clinical Studies Group. A randomised trial of radical radiotherapy in pT1G3 NXM0 bladder cancer (MRC BS06). *Proc Am Soc Clin Oncol.* 2005;23:Abstract 4505.
12. Lamm DL, Blumenstein BA, Crissman JD, et al. Maintenance bacillus Calmette-Guerin immunotherapy for recurrent TA, T1 and carcinoma in situ transitional cell carcinoma of the bladder: a randomized Southwest Oncology Group Study. *J Urol.* 2000;163:1124–1129.

13. Sylvester RJ, van der MA, Lamm DL. Intravesical bacillus Calmette-Guerin reduces the risk of progression in patients with superficial bladder cancer: a meta-analysis of the published results of randomized clinical trials. *J Urol.* 2002;168:1964–1970.

14. Herr HW, Schwalb DM, Zhang ZF, et al. Intravesical bacillus Calmette-Guerin therapy prevents tumor progression and death from superficial bladder cancer: ten-year follow-up of a prospective randomized trial. *J Clin Oncol.* 1995;13:1404–1408.

15. Lamm DL. BCG immunotherapy for transitional-cell carcinoma in situ of the bladder. *Oncology.* 1995;9:947–952, 955; discussion 955–965.

16. de Reijke TM, Kurth KH, Sylvester RJ, et al. Bacillus Calmette-Guerin versus epirubicin for primary, secondary or concurrent carcinoma in situ of the bladder: results of a European Organization for the Research and Treatment of Cancer—Genito-Urinary Group Phase III Trial (30906). *J Urol.* 2005;173:405–409.

17. Lamm DL, Blumenstein BA, Crawford ED, et al. A randomized trial of intravesical doxorubicin and immunotherapy with bacille Calmette-Guerin for transitional-cell carcinoma of the bladder. *N Engl J Med.* 1991;325:1205–1209.

18. Martinez-Pineiro JA, Jimenez Leon J, Martinez-Pineiro L Jr., et al. Bacillus Calmette-Guerin versus doxorubicin versus thiotepa: a randomized prospective study in 202 patients with superficial bladder cancer. *J Urol.* 1990;143:502–506.

19. Shelley MD, Court JB, Kynaston H, et al. Intravesical bacillus Calmette-Guerin versus mitomycin C for Ta and T1 bladder cancer. *Cochrane Database Syst Rev.* 2003:CD003231.

20. Lamm DL. Efficacy and safety of bacille Calmette-Guerin immunotherapy in superficial bladder cancer. *Clin Infect Dis.* 2000;31(suppl 3):S86–S90.

21. Pawinski A, Sylvester R, Kurth KH, et al. A combined analysis of European Organization for Research and Treatment of Cancer, and Medical Research Council randomized clinical trials for the prophylactic treatment of stage TaT1 bladder cancer. European Organization for Research and Treatment of Cancer Genitourinary Tract Cancer Cooperative Group and the Medical Research Council Working Party on Superficial Bladder Cancer. *J Urol.* 1996;156:1934–1940; discussion 1940–1941.

22. Schrag D, Hsieh LJ, Rabbani F, et al. Adherence to surveillance among patients with superficial bladder cancer. *J Natl Cancer Inst.* 2003;95:588–597.

CHAPTER 4

Muscle-Invasive Bladder Cancer

■ Overview

■ Radical cystectomy with pelvic lymph node dissection is the standard approach to the management of patients with bladder tumors that infiltrate the muscularis propria.

■ Organ-sparing procedures may be possible in a select subgroup of patients.

■ Other indications for radical cystectomy:
  ● Superficial bladder tumors that have failed conservative therapy
  ● Recurrent high-grade T1 disease
  ● Symptoms or bleeding related to bladder pathology that cannot be managed conservatively

■ Radical Cystectomy

■ A radical cystectomy involves a wide resection of the bladder with all of the perivesical fat and tissue in an attempt to achieve negative margins.

■ A prostatectomy is also performed in men; in women, the urethra, uterus, fallopian tubes, ovaries, anterior vaginal wall, and surrounding fascia are removed.

■ A standard pelvic lymph node dissection includes removal of the distal common iliac, external iliac, obturator, and hypogastric nodes.

■ Urinary flow can be directed through either a conduit diversion or a continent reservoir.
  ● *Conduit (incontinent) diversions*: Urine is drained directly from the ureters to the skin surface with no internal reservoir. A segment of bowel is used to bridge the gap between the ureters and the skin.

• *Continent reservoirs*: Include continent stomas, in which patients self-catheterize at regular intervals, and internal, orthotopic neobladders, with which patients may void in the natural position.

■ Prognosis After Radical Cystectomy

▩ Prognosis after surgery for bladder cancer depends on pathologic stage.

▩ In a large single-center series of 1,054 patients treated with radical cystectomy for bladder cancer, the 5-year disease-free survival rate for patients with node-negative organ-confined disease exceeded 80% but dropped to 62–78% for patients with extravesical disease (pT3) and 50% for patients with invasion of local organs (pT4). Patients with nodal disease had worse outcomes, with a 5-year disease-free survival rate of 35%.[1]

▩ A multinational database has been developed and utilized to construct a nomogram in an attempt to better estimate risk of progression/death in individual patients undergoing cystectomy.[2] This nomogram is available at www.nomograms.org.

▩ Several retrospective studies have correlated the extent of lymphadenectomy (and pathologic review) with improved survival.

  • In an analysis exploring the association between surgical/pathologic variables and survival in a series of 637 patients, improved survival and decreased local recurrence were associated with an increased number of lymph nodes removed (and examined by the pathologist). The association was observed in patients with both node-negative and node-positive disease. The 5-year survival rate for patients with 0–6, 6–10, 11–14, and >14 lymph nodes examined was 33%, 44%, 73%, and 79%, respectively.[3]

  • Similar results were reported from a second study analyzing Surveillance Epidemiology and End Results (SEER) data on 1,923 patients who underwent radical cystectomy.[4]

■ Perioperative Chemotherapy for Bladder Cancer

■ Given the poor outcomes in patients with extravesical extension and/or regional lymph node involvement, several (mostly underpowered) studies have explored the use of perioperative chemotherapy in an attempt to eradicate micrometastases and improve the likelihood of cure.

■ Neoadjuvant therapy

   ● Refers to administration of chemotherapy prior to definitive local therapy (e.g., surgery or radiation) in an attempt to eradicate micrometastases.

   ● There are both advantages and disadvantages with a neoadjuvant approach (see **Table 4.1**).

   ● One advantage of the neoadjuvant approach is the opportunity to evaluate the response of the primary tumor, which is of prognostic significance. In a study of patients treated with neoadjuvant cisplatin-based therapy followed by definitive surgery, patients with a major pathologic response (p stage <T2) had a 5-year survival of 75%, in contrast to 20% for the remaining nonresponding patients (p stage ≥T2).[5]

   ● Several randomized trials have explored neoadjuvant chemotherapy in bladder cancer (see **Table 4.2**). Many

Table 4.1   Advantages of Neoadjuvant and Adjuvant Systemic Therapy in Bladder Cancer

Advantages of Neoadjuvant Approach	Advantages of Adjuvant Approach
■ Systemic therapy can be initiated sooner.	■ Decision to use chemotherapy is based on more precise pathologic staging rather than clinical staging.
■ Treatment is better tolerated prior to surgery than in the postoperative setting.	■ Prevents delay of potentially "curative" surgery.
■ Response of primary tumor can be assessed, which is of prognostic significance.	

Table 4.2 Randomized Trials of Neoadjuvant Chemotherapy

Reference	n	Chemotherapy	Primary Treatment	Survival Benefit?
Hall[6]	975	CMV	RT/Cyst/Both	Yes
Grossman et al.[7]	317	MVAC	Cyst	Yes
Malmstrom et al.[8]	325	C + A	RT/Cyst	Yes*
Malmstrom et al.[9]	317	C + M	Cyst	No
Martinez-Pineiro et al.[10]	122	C	Cyst	No
Shipley et al.[11]	123	CMV	C + RT/Cyst	No
Cortesi[12]	171	MVEC	Cyst	No

M, methotrexate; C, cisplatin; V, vinblastine; A, doxorubicin; 5-FU, 5-fluorouracil; E, epirubicin; Cyst, cystectomy; RT, radiation therapy.

*Benefit for subset with T3–T4.

of these trials failed to show a benefit for chemotherapy. However, these studies suffered from small sample size, suboptimal chemotherapy, premature closure, or inadequate follow-up time. Recently, well-designed trials utilizing effective chemotherapeutic regimens have shifted the standard of care in muscle-invasive disease toward the use of neoadjuvant chemotherapy:

- A United States Intergroup Study (INT-008) randomized patients with muscle-invasive bladder cancer to radical cystectomy alone (154 patients) compared with three cycles of MVAC (methotrexate, vinblastine, doxorubicin, cisplatin) followed by radical cystectomy (153 patients).[7] Neoadjuvant chemotherapy was associated with a higher rate of complete pathologic response (38% compared with 15%, $p < 0.001$). At a median follow-up of 8.7 years, improvements in median survival (77 months compared with 46 months, $p = 0.06$) and 5-year survival rate (57% compared with 43%, $p = 0.06$) favored the neoadjuvant arm. Approximately one-third of patients treated with MVAC developed grade ≥ 3 hematologic or gastrointestinal toxicity; however, there were no treatment-related deaths, and neoadjuvant chemotherapy did not adversely affect the ability to proceed with radical cystectomy or increase adverse events related to surgery.

- A Medical Research Council (MRC)/European Organization for Research and Treatment of Cancer (EORTC) trial randomized 976 patients with muscle-invasive disease to neoadjuvant cisplatin, methotrexate, plus vinblastine (CMV; 491 patients) or no neoadjuvant chemotherapy (485 patients).[13] Management of the primary tumor involved cystectomy, radiation therapy, or both. At a median follow-up of approximately 7 years, an improvement in survival was observed for patients who received neoadjuvant chemotherapy ($p = 0.048$; hazard ratio [HR] = 0.85; 95% confidence interval [CI] 0.72–1.0).[14]

- A meta-analysis has confirmed a significant survival benefit associated with platinum-based combination neoadjuvant chemotherapy (HR = 0.86, 95% CI 0.77–0.95, $p = 0.003$), with an absolute improvement in survival of 5% at 5 years.[15]

- Adjuvant therapy
  - Refers to administration of chemotherapy after definitive local therapy (e.g., surgery or radiation) in an attempt to eradicate micrometastases.
  - There are both advantages and disadvantages with an adjuvant approach (see Table 4.1).
  - A particular advantage of adjuvant therapy is the opportunity to make the decision to pursue perioperative therapy based on more precise pathologic staging information. This is important because there is a significant discrepancy between clinical staging (based on exam under anesthesia and TURBT) and pathologic staging (based on pathologic review of the cystectomy

specimen). For example, a patient with a clinical T2 tumor that proves to be a pathologic T2 tumor after cystectomy has a favorable prognosis, and perioperative chemotherapy would likely provide only a minor benefit. However, a patient with a clinical T2 tumor that is really a pathologic T3N1 tumor has a poorer prognosis and substantially more to gain by integrating perioperative chemotherapy.

- At least seven randomized trials have evaluated the role of adjuvant chemotherapy following cystectomy (see **Table 4.3**). These trials have all been underpowered and/or closed early due to poor accrual, and/or utilized suboptimal chemotherapy. Nonetheless, three trials did suggest a survival benefit with adjuvant chemotherapy. The methodologic flaws of these trials have led many to question the validity of these results, however.

Table 4.3 Randomized Trials of Adjuvant Chemotherapy

Reference	n	Chemotherapy	Primary Treatment	Survival Benefit?
Skinner et al.[16]	91	CAP	Cyst	Yes
Stockle et al.[17]	49	MVA(E)C	Cyst	Yes
Studer et al.[18]	77	C	Cyst	No
Bono et al.[19]	83	CM	Cyst	No
Freiha et al.[20]	50	CMV	Cyst	No
Paz-Ares	142	GCP	Cyst	Yes
Cognetti	194	GC	Cyst	No

M, methotrexate; C, cisplatin; V, vinblastine; A, doxorubicin; 5-FU, 5-fluorouracil; E, epirubicin; G, gemcitabine; P, paclitaxel; Cyst, cystectomy.

Source: Cognetti F, Ruggeri EM, Feliciet A, et al., *J Clin Oncol.* 2008;26 (suppl abstr 5023).

Paz-Ares LG, Solsona E, Esteban E, et al., *J Clin Oncol.* 2010 (suppl: abstr LBA 4518).

- Perioperative chemotherapy recommendations/choice of regimen
  - The data support the use of cisplatin-based combination chemotherapy regimens (particularly MVAC or CMV) as neoadjuvant therapy for patients with muscle-invasive bladder cancer. For patients with metastatic disease, the combination of gemcitabine plus cisplatin has been shown to result in comparable response proportions and overall survival when compared with MVAC, but with less toxicity.[21] Although definitive randomized trials exploring perioperative gemcitabine plus cisplatin have not been performed, many experts have extrapolated the results from a trial showing similar efficacy between gemcitabine plus cisplatin and MVAC in patients with metastatic bladder cancer and adopted this regimen for use in the perioperative setting. Approximately 3 months of neoadjuvant chemotherapy are administered followed by cystectomy.
  - Given the less compelling data for adjuvant chemotherapy, divergent opinions exist regarding the current standard of care. Most U.S. oncologists extrapolate the data from the neoadjuvant trials and employ cisplatin-based combination adjuvant chemotherapy for patients with pT3–4 or node-positive (N1) bladder cancer. Similar to the neoadjuvant setting, the most commonly employed regimens are 3 months of MVAC or gemcitabine plus cisplatin. An EORTC trial is currently randomizing patients with pT3–4 and/or node-positive disease to immediate cisplatin-based chemotherapy (MVAC or gemcitabine/cisplatin) or similar chemotherapy at the time of relapse in an effort to definitively evaluate the role of adjuvant chemotherapy.

■ Bladder-Sparing Approaches for Muscle-Invasive Bladder Cancer

- Several approaches have been explored in an effort to avoid complete removal of the bladder in patients with invasive bladder cancer, including partial cystectomy, radiation therapy, and concurrent chemoradiation.

- Partial cystectomy
  - Refers to removal of the segment of bladder involved with tumor. This approach also allows pelvic lymph node dissection.
  - Although the overall results with partial cystectomy appear inferior to radical cystectomy, particularly with regard to local recurrence, patients meeting the following criteria may be best suited for this approach:[22]
    - Solitary tumor
    - Lack of involvement of the bladder neck or trigone
    - Ability to completely resect the tumor with a 2-cm margin
    - Absence of carcinoma in situ
    - Adequate bladder capacity
- Radiation therapy
  - Radiation therapy as definitive treatment for bladder cancer is commonly employed in patients who are not surgical candidates.
  - Although no randomized studies have been performed, this approach appears inferior to radical cystectomy, with 5-year survival rates of approximately 20–40%.[23]
- Combined modality therapy
  - Several trials have explored TURBT followed by concurrent chemoradiation as a bladder-sparing approach.
  - Although no large randomized trials have directly compared radiation therapy alone with concurrent chemoradiation as definitive therapy for bladder cancer, a National Cancer Institute of Canada trial did evaluate the role of radiation therapy given with or without concurrent cisplatin as definitive therapy or as precystectomy therapy. (Patients and their physicians selected either definitive radiotherapy or precystectomy radiotherapy.)[24] For the entire cohort (99 patients), the addition of cisplatin to radiation therapy was associated with a significant improvement in local control but not an improvement in overall survival.
  - A series of trials have explored a variety of combined modality regimens as bladder preservation therapy (see **Table 4.4**).

Table 4.4   Selected Trials of Combined Modality Bladder-Sparing Therapy

Reference	n	Adjuvant/ Neoadjuvant Chemotherapy	Radiation Therapy	Radiation Sensitizer	Survival Rate	Intact Bladder
Tester et al.[25]	42	None	Daily	C	52% 5-yr	NA
Tester et al.[26]	91	Neoadjuvant CMV	Daily	C	62% 4-yr	44% 4-yr
Kaufman et al.[27]	34	None	Hypofractionated	C + 5-FU	83% 3-yr	66% 3-yr
Hagan et al.[28]	52	Adjuvant CMV	Twice daily	C	61% 3-yr	48% 3-yr

M, methotrexate; C, cisplatin; V, vinblastine; 5-FU, 5-fluorouracil.

- There have been no randomized trials comparing the results of bladder-sparing therapy with radical cystectomy. Compared with historical controls, the use of a combined modality approach in appropriately selected patients has yielded similar outcomes. Five-year survival rates of 50–60% have been reported, with approximately 70% of those patients maintaining an intact bladder.[29]
- In an analysis of quality of life in patients treated with bladder preservation, the majority of patients with an intact bladder preserved normal bladder function, and low rates of bowel symptoms and urinary incontinence were reported.[30]
- When considering combined modality therapy as a bladder preservation approach (in patients who are otherwise medically fit for cystectomy), patients should be carefully selected for predictors of favorable outcome, including:
  - Clinical stage T2 disease amenable to complete resection by TURBT
  - Absence of ureteral obstruction
  - Ability to receive cisplatin-based chemotherapy
  - Absence of multifocal disease or carcinoma in situ

■ References

1. Stein JP, Lieskovsky G, Cote R, et al. Radical cystectomy in the treatment of invasive bladder cancer: long-term results in 1,054 patients. *J Clin Oncol.* 2001;19:666–675.
2. Bochner BH, Kattan MW, Vora KC. Postoperative nomogram predicting risk of recurrence after radical cystectomy for bladder cancer. *J Clin Oncol.* 2006;24:3967–3972.
3. Herr HW. Extent of surgery and pathology evaluation has an impact on bladder cancer outcomes after radical cystectomy. *Urology.* 2003;61:105–108.
4. Konety BR, Joslyn SA. Factors influencing aggressive therapy for bladder cancer: an analysis of data from the SEER program. *J Urol.* 2003;170:1765–1771.
5. Splinter TA, Scher HI, Denis L, et al. The prognostic value of the pathological response to combination chemotherapy before cystectomy in patients with invasive bladder cancer. European Organization for Research on Treatment of Cancer—Genitourinary Group. *J Urol.* 1992;147:606–608.

6. Hall R. Updated results of a randomised controlled trial of neoadjuvant cisplatin (C), methotrexate (M) and vinblastine (V) chemotherapy for muscle-invasive bladder cancer (abstract 710). *Proc Am Soc Clin Oncol.* 2002;21:178a.

7. Grossman HB, Natale RB, Tangen CM, et al. Neoadjuvant chemotherapy plus cystectomy compared with cystectomy alone for locally advanced bladder cancer. *N Engl J Med.* 2003;349:859–866.

8. Malmstrom PU, Rintala E, Wahlqvist R, et al. Five-year followup of a prospective trial of radical cystectomy and neoadjuvant chemotherapy: Nordic Cystectomy Trial I. The Nordic Cooperative Bladder Cancer Study Group. *J Urol.* 1996;155:1903–1906.

9. Malmstrom PU, Rintala E, Wahlqvist R, et al. Neoadjuvant cisplatin-methotrexate chemotherapy of invasive bladder cancer: Nordic cystectomy trial 2: XIVth Congress of the European Association of Urology (abstract 238). *Eur Urol.* 1999;35(suppl 2):60.

10. Martinez-Pineiro JA, Gonzalez Martin M, Arocena F, et al. Neoadjuvant cisplatin chemotherapy before radical cystectomy in invasive transitional cell carcinoma of the bladder: a prospective randomized phase III study. *J Urol.* 1995;153:964–973.

11. Shipley WU, Winter KA, Kaufman DS, et al. Phase III trial of neoadjuvant chemotherapy in patients with invasive bladder cancer treated with selective bladder preservation by combined radiation therapy and chemotherapy: initial results of Radiation Therapy Oncology Group 89-03. *J Clin Oncol.* 1998;16:3576–3583.

12. Cortesi E. Neoadjuvant treatment for locally advanced bladder cancer: a prospective randomized clinical trial (abstract 623). *Proc Am Soc Clin Oncol.* 1995;14:237.

13. Neoadjuvant cisplatin, methotrexate, and vinblastine chemotherapy for muscle-invasive bladder cancer: a randomised controlled trial. International collaboration of trialists. *Lancet.* 1999;354:533–540.

14. Hall RR. Updated results of a randomised controlled trial of neoadjuvant cisplatin (C), methotrexate (M) and vinblastine (V) chemotherapy for muscle-invasive bladder cancer. *Proc Am Soc Clin Oncol.* 2002;21:Abstract 710.

15. Neoadjuvant chemotherapy in invasive bladder cancer: update of a systematic review and meta-analysis of individual patient data advanced bladder cancer (ABC) meta-analysis collaboration. *Eur Urol.* 2005;48:202–205; discussion 205–206.

16. Skinner DG, Daniels JR, Russell CA, et al. The role of adjuvant chemotherapy following cystectomy for invasive

bladder cancer: a prospective comparative trial. *J Urol.* 1991;145:459–464; discussion 464–467.

17. Stockle M, Meyenburg W, Wellek S, et al. Advanced bladder cancer (stages pT3b, pT4a, pN1 and pN2): improved survival after radical cystectomy and 3 adjuvant cycles of chemotherapy. Results of a controlled prospective study. *J Urol.* 1992;148:302–306; discussion 306–307.

18. Studer UE, Bacchi M, Biedermann C, et al. Adjuvant cisplatin chemotherapy following cystectomy for bladder cancer: results of a prospective randomized trial. *J Urol.* 1994;152:81–84.

19. Bono AV, Benvenuti C, Reali L, et al. Adjuvant chemotherapy in advanced bladder cancer. Italian Uro-Oncologic Cooperative Group. *Prog Clin Biol Res.* 1989;303:533–540.

20. Freiha F, Reese J, Torti FM. A randomized trial of radical cystectomy versus radical cystectomy plus cisplatin, vinblastine and methotrexate chemotherapy for muscle invasive bladder cancer. *J Urol.* 1996;155:495–499; discussion 499–500.

21. von der Maase H, Hansen SW, Roberts JT, et al. Gemcitabine and cisplatin versus methotrexate, vinblastine, doxorubicin, and cisplatin in advanced or metastatic bladder cancer: results of a large, randomized, multinational, multicenter, phase III study. *J Clin Oncol.* 2000;18:3068–3077.

22. Kassouf W, Swanson D, Kamat AM, et al. Partial cystectomy for muscle invasive urothelial carcinoma of the bladder: a contemporary review of the M. D. Anderson Cancer Center experience. *J Urol.* 2006;175:2058–2062.

23. Gospodarowicz MK, Quilty PM, Scalliet P, et al. The place of radiation therapy as definitive treatment of bladder cancer. *Int J Urol.* 1995;2(suppl 2):41–48.

24. Coppin CM, Gospodarowicz MK, James K, et al. Improved local control of invasive bladder cancer by concurrent cisplatin and preoperative or definitive radiation. The National Cancer Institute of Canada Clinical Trials Group. *J Clin Oncol.* 1996;14:2901–2907.

25. Tester W, Porter A, Asbell S, et al. Combined modality program with possible organ preservation for invasive bladder carcinoma: results of RTOG protocol 85-12. *Int J Radiat Oncol Biol Phys.* 1993;25:783–790.

26. Tester W, Caplan R, Heaney J, et al. Neoadjuvant combined modality program with selective organ preservation for invasive bladder cancer: results of Radiation Therapy Oncology Group phase II trial 8802. *J Clin Oncol.* 1996;14:119–126.

27. Kaufman DS, Winter KA, Shipley WU, et al. The initial results in muscle-invading bladder cancer of RTOG 95-06: phase I/II trial of transurethral surgery plus radiation therapy with concurrent cisplatin and 5-fluorouracil followed by

selective bladder preservation or cystectomy depending on the initial response. *Oncologist.* 2000;5:471–476.

28. Hagan MP, Winter KA, Kaufman DS, et al. RTOG 97-06: initial report of a phase I-II trial of selective bladder conservation using TURBT, twice-daily accelerated irradiation sensitized with cisplatin, and adjuvant MCV combination chemotherapy. *Int J Radiat Oncol Biol Phys.* 2003;57:665–672.

29. Michaelson MD, Shipley WU, Heney NM, et al. Selective bladder preservation for muscle-invasive transitional cell carcinoma of the urinary bladder. *Br J Cancer.* 2004;90: 578–581.

30. Zietman AL, Sacco D, Skowronski U, et al. Organ conservation in invasive bladder cancer by transurethral resection, chemotherapy and radiation: results of a urodynamic and quality of life study on long-term survivors. *J Urol.* 2003;170:1772–1776.

Urothelial Carcinoma of the Ureter and Renal Pelvis

■ Overview

▪ Transitional cell carcinomas of the renal pelvis and ureters ("upper tract") account for approximately 10% of cancers of the urothelial tract.

▪ Less than 5% of all renal tumors are transitional cell carcinomas.

▪ In Balkan countries, the incidence of transitional cell carcinoma of the renal pelvis is much higher, accounting for approximately 50% of renal tumors, due to an endemic familial nephropathy.

▪ Multifocal tumors (synchronous or metachronous) are often present in patients with urothelial carcinoma, and patients with upper tract tumors are at risk for the development of cancers in the bladder and vice versa.

■ Diagnosis, Staging, and Prognosis

▪ Hematuria is the most common sign of a cancer of the upper urothelial tract.

▪ Flank pain may occur due to ureteral obstruction.

▪ The diagnosis of a cancer of the ureter or pelvis is often suggested by an abnormal CT scan or intravenous pyelogram (IVP). CT urography offers a detailed view of the upper urinary tract and has largely replaced standard IVP.

▪ Ureteroscopy allows direct visualization of the upper urinary tract. Biopsies of abnormal sites are then obtained to confirm the diagnosis.

▪ Routine staging should include a chest x-ray, a CT scan of the abdomen, and a bone scan if there are symptoms suggestive of bone metastases or an elevated alkaline phosphatase level.

- The TNM staging system for cancers of the upper urothelial tract is similar to the staging system for bladder cancers (see **Tables 5.1** and **5.2**).
- The prognosis for a patient with transitional cell carcinoma of the upper urinary tract is associated with the grade and stage of the tumor (see **Table 5.3**).

Table 5.1   Staging of Renal Pelvis and Ureteral Cancers

T Stage (Primary Tumor)	
Tis	Carcinoma in situ
Ta	Papillary noninvasive carcinoma
T1	Tumor invades subepithelial connective tissue
T2	Tumor invades the muscularis
T3	(For renal pelvis only) Tumor invades beyond muscularis into peripelvic fat or the renal parenchyma (For ureter only) Tumor invades beyond muscularis into periureteric fat
T4	Tumor invades adjacent organs, or through the kidney into the perinephric fat
N Stage (Lymph Nodes)	
N0	No regional lymph node metastases are detected
N1	Metastasis in a single lymph node, 2 cm in greatest diameter
N2	Metastasis in a single lymph node, more than 2 cm but not more than 5 cm in greatest diameter; or multiple lymph nodes, none more than 5 cm in greatest diameter
N3	Metastasis in a lymph node more than 5 cm in greatest diameter
M Stage (Metastases)	
M0	No distant metastasis
M1	Distant metastasis

Source: Used with the permission of the American Joint Committee on Cancer (AJCC), Chicago, Illinois. The original source for this material is the *AJCC Cancer Staging Manual,* Seventh Edition (2010), published by Springer Science and Business Media LLC, www.springer.com.

Table 5.2   Renal Pelvis and Ureteral Cancer Stage Groupings

Stage Grouping	T Stage	N Stage	M Stage
0a	Ta	N0	M0
0is	Tis	N0	M0
I	T1	N0	M0
II	T2	N0	M0
III	T3	N0	M0
IV	T4	N0	M0
	Any T	N1–3	M0
	Any T	Any N	M1

Source: Used with the permission of the American Joint Committee on Cancer (AJCC), Chicago, Illinois. The original source for this material is the *AJCC Cancer Staging Manual,* Seventh Edition (2010), published by Springer Science and Business Media LLC, www.springer.com.

Table 5.3   Prognosis of Patients with Transitional Cell Carcinoma of the Upper Urothelial Tract

Stage Rate	5-Year Disease-Specific Survival
Carcinoma in situ	95%
Localized	89%
Regional metastases	63%
Distant metastases	17%

Source: Data derived from Munoz & Ellison.[1]

■ Treatment of Localized Disease

- Nephroureterectomy (removal of the entire ureter and kidney) is the procedure of choice for localized transitional cell carcinomas of the upper urothelial tract. This is due to the high rate of recurrent tumors when a portion of the upper urinary tract is left intact.[2] Laparoscopic approaches have been associated with less morbidity than traditional open procedures. Although acceptable antitumor outcomes have also been reported, most series have been limited to single-center experience with short follow-up.[3]

- Kidney-sparing approaches have been utilized and may be acceptable for some patients (e.g., bilateral tumors, solitary kidney, low ureteral lesion).
- Endoscopic management may be appropriate for focal low-grade lesions.[4]

■ Treatment of Locally Advanced Disease

- There have been no randomized trials exploring the benefit of postoperative radiation therapy for patients with locally advanced (e.g., T3/T4 or N1) disease. Retrospective series suggest an improvement in local control with radiation therapy, but the impact on survival remains uncertain.[5]
- There have been no randomized trials exploring the benefit of adjuvant chemotherapy in patients with locally advanced transitional cell carcinoma of the upper urinary tract. Several retrospective trials have suggested a survival benefit, including a study exploring concurrent chemoradiation.[6–8] A single-arm prospective trial has demonstrated the safety of adjuvant paclitaxel and carboplatin, with a suggestion of an improvement in outcomes compared with historical controls.[9]
- The benefit of adjuvant radiation, chemotherapy, or chemoradiation after resection of locally advanced transitional cell carcinoma of the upper urothelial tract remains unproven. However, randomized trials may never be performed in this relatively rare population, and decisions regarding treatment should be individualized based on a discussion of the available data and patient preferences regarding treatment.

■ Treatment of Metastatic Disease

- The treatment of metastatic transitional cell carcinoma of the upper urothelial tract is identical to the treatment of metastatic transitional cell carcinoma of the bladder (see Chapter 6).

■ References

1. Munoz JJ, Ellison LM. Upper tract urothelial neoplasms: incidence and survival during the last 2 decades. *J Urol.* 2000;164:1523–1525.
2. Strong DW, Pearse HD. Recurrent urothelial tumors following surgery for transitional cell carcinoma of the upper urinary tract. *Cancer.* 1976;38:2173–2183.
3. Gill IS, Sung GT, Hobart MG, et al. Laparoscopic radical nephroureterectomy for upper tract transitional cell carcinoma: the Cleveland Clinic experience. *J Urol.* 2000; 164:1513–1522.
4. Daneshmand S, Quek ML, Huffman JL. Endoscopic management of upper urinary tract transitional cell carcinoma: long-term experience. *Cancer.* 2003;98:55–60.
5. Cozad SC, Smalley SR, Austenfeld M, et al. Adjuvant radiotherapy in high stage transitional cell carcinoma of the renal pelvis and ureter. *Int J Radiat Oncol Biol Phys.* 1992;24:743–745.
6. Czito B, Zietman A, Kaufman D, et al. Adjuvant radiotherapy with and without concurrent chemotherapy for locally advanced transitional cell carcinoma of the renal pelvis and ureter. *J Urol.* 2004;172:1271–1275.
7. Kwak C, Lee SE, Jeong IG, et al. Adjuvant systemic chemotherapy in the treatment of patients with invasive transitional cell carcinoma of the upper urinary tract. *Urology.* 2006;68:53–57.
8. Michael M, Tannock IF, Czaykowski PM, et al. Adjuvant chemotherapy for high-risk urothelial transitional cell carcinoma: the Princess Margaret Hospital experience. *Br J Urol.* 1998;82:366–372.
9. Bamias A, Deliveliotis C, Fountzilas G, et al. Adjuvant chemotherapy with paclitaxel and carboplatin in patients with advanced carcinoma of the upper urinary tract: a study by the Hellenic Cooperative Oncology Group. *J Clin Oncol.* 2004;22:2150–2154.

Metastatic Urothelial Carcinoma

■ Overview

■ Approximately 25% of patients with bladder cancer present de novo with metastatic disease.

■ Approximately 50% of patients undergoing radical cystectomy for muscle-invasive bladder cancer develop distant metastases.

■ The term *urothelial carcinoma,* rather than *bladder cancer,* is used for the remainder of the chapter because regardless of the site of origin within the urothelial tract, once metastatic, there is no difference in the chemotherapeutic regimens employed.

■ The median survival for patients with metastatic urothelial carcinoma is approximately 14 months; however, urothelial carcinoma is a chemosensitive neoplasm and outcomes are extremely heterogeneous depending on the distribution of baseline prognostic factors and response to treatment.

■ MVAC: Historical Perspective

■ The MVAC regimen was developed in the 1980s utilizing a combination of the most active single agents of the time—methotrexate, vinblastine, Adriamycin (doxorubicin), and cisplatin.

■ In the landmark pilot trial, 24 patients with advanced or unresectable urothelial carcinoma were treated with MVAC.[1] Responses were observed in 71% (95% CI 53–89%) of those treated, with complete clinical responses in 50% (95% CI 30–70%).

■ Several other investigators confirmed the activity of MVAC in larger trials, with slightly lower overall and complete response rates.

- Subsequent randomized trials proved MVAC superior to single-agent cisplatin and the combination regimen CISCA (cisplatin, cyclophosphamide, and doxorubicin), and MVAC was adopted as a standard of care (see **Table 6.1**).
- MVAC was limited by toxicity: treatment-related deaths (2–4%), febrile neutropenia (20–30%), mucositis (10–20%), renal impairment, hearing loss, and peripheral neuropathy.
- Attempts to improve MVAC have included dose-dense administration with granulocyte colony-stimulating factor support. A randomized trial of dose-dense MVAC versus conventional MVAC in patients with metastatic bladder cancer conducted by the EORTC resulted in similar outcomes (see Table 6.1).[5] With longer follow-up (a median follow-up of 7.3 years), 24.6% of patients on the dose-dense arm were alive compared with 13.2% on the standard dose arm, suggesting a subset of patients may benefit from this approach.[10]

■ Newer Combination Regimens in Metastatic Urothelial Carcinoma

- Trials evaluating single-agent activity with gemcitabine and the taxanes demonstrated promising activity and led to the development of multiagent regimens incorporating these drugs (see Table 6.1).
- A landmark phase III trial randomized 405 patients with metastatic urothelial carcinoma to gemcitabine plus cisplatin (GC) versus MVAC.[6] Although this trial was not designed as a noninferiority trial, the overall survival was similar on both arms (HR 1.04; 95% CI 0.82–1.32; $p = 0.75$). More patients on the GC arm completed all six cycles of therapy. As expected, the GC arm was associated with a favorable toxicity profile: toxic death rate (1% versus 3%), neutropenic fever (14% versus 2%), neutropenic sepsis (12% versus 1%), grade 3/4 mucositis (22% versus 1%), and alopecia (55% versus 11%). Based on this trial, gemcitabine plus cisplatin has become a widely utilized treatment standard for metastatic urothelial carcinoma.

Table 6.1 Randomized Trials in Metastatic Urothelial Carcinoma

Reference	Regimens	n	Overall Response Rate	Median Survival (months)	p
Loehrer et al.[2]	MVAC Cisplatin	246	36% 11%	12.5 8.2	<0.0002
Logothetis et al.[3]	MVAC CISCA	110	65% 46%	12.6 10	<0.05
Siefker-Radtke et al.[4]	MVAC FAP	169	59% 42%	12.5 12.5	0.17
Sternberg et al.[5]	MVAC HD-MVAC	263	58% 72%	14.1 15.5	0.122
Von der Maase et al.[6]	MVAC Gemcitabine + cisplatin	408	46% 50%	14.8 13.8	0.746
Bamias et al.[7]	MVAC Docetaxel + cisplatin	220	54% 37%	14.2 9.3	0.025
Dreicer et al.[8]	MVAC Paclitaxel + carboplatin	85*	40% 28%	14.2 13.8	0.41
Bellmunt et al.[9]	Gemcitabine + cisplatin Gemcitabine + cisplatin + paclitaxel	627	46% 57%	12.8 15.7	NS

MVAC, methotrexate, vinblastine, doxorubicin, cisplatin; CISCA, cyclophosphamide, cisplatin, doxorubicin; CMV, cisplatin, methotrexate, vinblastine; FAP, 5-fluorouracil, interferon-alfa-2b, cisplatin; HD-MVAC, high-dose MVAC; NS, not statistically significant.

*Trial closed early with only 85 patients.

- MVAC was associated with superior response rates and overall survival in a trial comparing MVAC with docetaxel plus cisplatin.
- A trial comparing gemcitabine plus cisplatin versus gemcitabine, cisplatin, plus paclitaxel conducted by the EORTC was reported at the American Society of Clinical Oncology (ASCO) annual meeting in 2007.[9] The improvement in median survival with the three-drug regimen did not reach statistical significance (15.7 months versus 12.8 months; $p = 0.10$).
- Based on randomized studies to date, GC and MVAC are acceptable standard regimens for patients with metastatic urothelial carcinoma.

■ Cisplatin-Ineligible Patients with Metastatic Urothelial Carcinoma

- Up to 40% of patients with urothelial carcinoma are ineligible for cisplatin-based therapy due to impaired renal function alone.[11] Therefore, carboplatin-based regimens have been extensively explored.
- No phase III trials have been designed to specifically address the equivalence of carboplatin and cisplatin in the treatment of metastatic urothelial carcinoma.
- The Eastern Cooperative Oncology Group initiated a phase III trial comparing MVAC with paclitaxel plus carboplatin. However, this study was terminated after 2.5 years due to poor accrual, leaving the results impossible to interpret.[8]
- Several randomized phase II studies have been completed, generally reporting higher overall and complete response rates with cisplatin-based regimens compared with carboplatin-based regimens (see **Table 6.2**).[12–14]
- A phase II/III study compared gemcitabine plus carboplatin with methotrexate, carboplatin, vinblastine in cisplatin-ineligible patients with metastatic bladder cancer.[15] This study revealed that both regimens were active in this patient population, although gemcitabine plus carboplatin was associated with less toxicity
- In patients with contraindications to cisplatin (e.g., creatinine clearance <60 mL/min or poor performance status), the doublets of gemcitabine plus carboplatin or paclitaxel

Table 6.2   Randomized Phase II Trials Comparing Cisplatin- and Carboplatin-Based Combinations in Metastatic Urothelial Carcinoma

Reference	Treatment Arms	Overall Response Rate	p	Complete Response Rate
Bellmunt et al.[12]	MVAC	52%	0.3	13%
	MCAVI	39%		0%
Petrioli et al.[13]	MVE-Cisplatin	71%	0.04	25%
	MVE-Carboplatin	41%		11%
Dogliotti et al.[14]	Gemcitabine + cisplatin	49%	NP	15%
	Gemcitabine + carboplatin	40%		2%

MVAC, methotrexate, vinblastine, doxorubicin, cisplatin; MCAVI, methotrexate, carboplatin, vinblastine; MVE, methotrexate, vinblastine, epirubicin; NP, not provided.

plus carboplatin are most commonly utilized based on phase II data suggesting activity and tolerability in this population of patients.[16–18]

■ Second-Line Chemotherapy in Metastatic Urothelial Carcinoma

- Multiple small phase II trials have been performed. Overall, the most active of these agents have shown response rates of approximately 10–30% (see **Table 6.3**).
- Currently, taxanes are most commonly utilized as second-line chemotherapy in patients previously treated with gemcitabine plus cisplatin or gemcitabine plus carboplatin.
- A phase III trial compared vinflunine (VFL) with placebo as second-line therapy in patients with metastatic urothelial carcinoma.[27] In the intent-to-treat population, the objective of a median 2-month survival advantage (6.9 months for VFL plus best supportive care [BSC] vs. 4.6 months for BSC; HR = 0.88; 95% CI 0.69–1.12) was achieved but did not reach statistical significance.

Table 6.3   Selected Second-Line Chemotherapy Trials in Metastatic Urothelial Carcinoma

Reference	Regimen	n	Overall Response Rate	95% Confidence Interval
Vaughn et al.[19]	Paclitaxel	31	10%	0–26%
McCaffrey et al.[20]	Docetaxel	30	13%	4–30%
Witte et al.[21]	Ifosfamide	56	20%	10–32%
Lorusso et al.[22]	Gemcitabine	35	20%	10–36%
Vaishampayan et al.[23]	Paclitaxel + carboplatin	44	16%	7–30%
Culine et al.[24]	Vinflunine	51	18%	8–31%
Galsky et al.[25]	Pemetrexed	13	8%	*
Sweeney et al.[26]	Pemetrexed	47	28%	16–43%

*90% upper limit = 29%.

■ Integration of Novel Agents in Urothelial Carcinoma

- Several pathways central to growth and progression of other solid tumors have been shown to be important in the pathogenesis of urothelial carcinoma in preclinical studies. The most extensively studied have involved tumor angiogenesis and signal transduction through the epidermal growth factor family of receptors.
- Single-arm phase II studies with inhibitors of endothelial growth factor receptor (EGFR) or human epidermal growth receptor 2 (HER-2) combined with standard chemotherapy have demonstrated safety and activity.[28,29] However, the contribution of the novel agents to these regimens is unclear in the absence of a randomized study.
- Studies exploring antiangiogenic agents are ongoing. The multitargeted tyrosine kinase inhibitor sunitinib, with

activity against the vascular endothelial growth factor receptor and the platelet-derived growth factor receptor, has shown modest single-agent activity in metastatic urothelial carcinoma and intriguing activity when combined with chemotherapy.[30–32]

▪ Based on a promising phase II study combining the antivascular endothelial growth factor antibody bevacizumab with gemcitabine plus cisplatin, a large randomized phase III trial exploring this regimen is ongoing.[33]

■ Prognostic Factors in Metastatic Urothelial Carcinoma

▪ Despite the generally poor prognosis for patients with metastatic urothelial carcinoma, outcomes are heterogeneous and a small proportion of patients do achieve prolonged progression-free survival.

▪ A landmark analysis evaluated predictors of outcome in 203 patients with advanced urothelial carcinoma treated with MVAC.[34] In a multivariate analysis, two factors were of independent prognostic significance: Karnofsky performance status ≤80% and visceral (lung, liver, or bone) metastases. The median survival for patients with zero, one, or two risk factors is shown in **Table 6.4**.

Table 6.4   Prognostic Factors in Advanced Urothelial Carcinoma

Number of Prognostic Factors	Median Survival (months)	5-Year Survival Rate	10-Year Survival Rate
0	33.0	33%	24%
1	13.4	11%	6%
2	9.2	0%	0%

Prognostic factors = Karnofsky performance status ≤80% and visceral (lung, liver, or bone) metastases.

Source: Adapted from Bajorin et al.[34]

■ Postchemotherapy Surgery in Metastatic Urothelial Carcinoma

■ Several analyses have demonstrated the benefit of postchemotherapy resection of residual disease after a response to chemotherapy in patients with advanced urothelial carcinoma.

■ In a retrospective evaluation, 50 of 203 patients with advanced urothelial carcinoma treated with MVAC underwent postchemotherapy resection of residual disease.[35] In 17 of 50 patients, no viable tumor was detected after pathologic analysis of the resected specimen, while 30 of 50 patients underwent complete resection of residual viable tumor. Approximately one in three of these patients were alive at 5 years. Optimal candidates for postchemotherapy surgery have prechemotherapy disease limited to the primary site and/or lymph nodes and achieve a near-complete response to chemotherapy.

■ References

1. Sternberg CN, Yagoda A, Scher HI, et al. Preliminary results of M-VAC (methotrexate, vinblastine, doxorubicin and cisplatin) for transitional cell carcinoma of the urothelium. *J Urol.* 1985;133:403–407.

2. Loehrer PJ Sr, Einhorn LH, Elson PJ, et al. A randomized comparison of cisplatin alone or in combination with methotrexate, vinblastine, and doxorubicin in patients with metastatic urothelial carcinoma: a cooperative group study. *J Clin Oncol.* 1992;10:1066–1073.

3. Logothetis CJ, Dexeus FH, Finn L, et al. A prospective randomized trial comparing MVAC and CISCA chemotherapy for patients with metastatic urothelial tumors. *J Clin Oncol.* 1990;8:1050–1055.

4. Siefker-Radtke AO, Millikan RE, Tu SM, et al. Phase III trial of fluorouracil, interferon alpha-2b, and cisplatin versus methotrexate, vinblastine, doxorubicin, and cisplatin in metastatic or unresectable urothelial cancer. *J Clin Oncol.* 2002; 20:1361–1367.

5. Sternberg CN, de Mulder PH, Schornagel JH, et al. Randomized phase III trial of high-dose-intensity methotrexate, vinblastine, doxorubicin, and cisplatin (MVAC) chemotherapy and recombinant human granulocyte colony-stimulating factor versus classic MVAC in advanced urothelial

tract tumors: European Organization for Research and Treatment of Cancer Protocol no. 30924. *J Clin Oncol.* 2001;19: 2638–2646.

6. von der Maase H, Hansen SW, Roberts JT, et al. Gemcitabine and cisplatin versus methotrexate, vinblastine, doxorubicin, and cisplatin in advanced or metastatic bladder cancer: results of a large, randomized, multinational, multicenter, phase III study. *J Clin Oncol.* 2000;18:3068–3077.

7. Bamias A, Aravantinos G, Deliveliotis C, et al. Docetaxel and cisplatin with granulocyte colony-stimulating factor (G-CSF) versus MVAC with G-CSF in advanced urothelial carcinoma: a multicenter, randomized, phase III study from the Hellenic Cooperative Oncology Group. *J Clin Oncol.* 2004;22:220–228.

8. Dreicer R, Manola J, Roth BJ, et al. Phase III trial of methotrexate, vinblastine, doxorubicin, and cisplatin versus carboplatin and paclitaxel in patients with advanced carcinoma of the urothelium. *Cancer.* 2004;100:1639–1645.

9. Bellmunt J, Von der Maase H, Mead GM, et al. Randomized phase III study comparing paclitaxel/cisplatin/gemcitabine and gemcitabine/cisplatin in patients with locally advanced or metastatic urothelial cancer without prior systemic therapy; EORTC30987/Intergroup Study. *Proc Am Soc Clin Oncol.* 2007;25:Abstract 5030.

10. Sternberg CN, de Mulder P, Schornagel JH, et al. Seven year update of an EORTC phase III trial of high-dose intensity M-VAC chemotherapy and G-CSF versus classic M-VAC in advanced urothelial tract tumours. *Eur J Cancer.* 2006;42:50–54.

11. Dash A, Galsky MD, Vickers AJ, et al. Impact of renal impairment on eligibility for adjuvant cisplatin-based chemotherapy in patients with urothelial carcinoma of the bladder. *Cancer.* 2006;107:506–513.

12. Bellmunt J, Ribas A, Eres N, et al. Carboplatin-based versus cisplatin-based chemotherapy in the treatment of surgically incurable advanced bladder carcinoma. *Cancer.* 1997;80: 1966–1972.

13. Petrioli R, Frediani B, Manganelli A, et al. Comparison between a cisplatin-containing regimen and a carboplatin-containing regimen for recurrent or metastatic bladder cancer patients. A randomized phase II study. *Cancer.* 1996;77: 344–351.

14. Dogliotti L, Carteni G, Siena S, et al. Gemcitabine plus cisplatin versus gemcitabine plus carboplatin as first-line chemotherapy in advanced transitional cell carcinoma of the urothelium: results of a randomized phase 2 trial. *Eur Urol.* 2007;52:134–141.

15. De Santis M, Bellmunt J, Mead G, et al. Randomized phase II/III trial assessing gemcitabine/carboplatin and methotrexate/carboplatin/vinblastine in patients with advanced urothelial cancer "unfit" for cisplatin-based chemotherapy: phase II—results of EORTC study 30986. *J Clin Oncol.* 2009;27:5634–5639.

16. Vaughn DJ, Manola J, Dreicer R, et al. Phase II study of paclitaxel plus carboplatin in patients with advanced carcinoma of the urothelium and renal dysfunction (E2896): a trial of the Eastern Cooperative Oncology Group. *Cancer.* 2002;95:1022–1027.

17. Linardou H, Aravantinos G, Efstathiou E, et al. Gemcitabine and carboplatin combination as first-line treatment in elderly patients and those unfit for cisplatin-based chemotherapy with advanced bladder carcinoma: phase II study of the Hellenic Cooperative Oncology Group. *Urology.* 2004;64:479–484.

18. Galsky MD, Iasonos A, Mironov S, et al. Phase II trial of dose-dense doxorubicin plus gemcitabine followed by paclitaxel plus carboplatin in patients with advanced urothelial carcinoma and impaired renal function. *Cancer.* 2007;109:549–555.

19. Vaughn DJ, Broome CM, Hussain M, et al. Phase II trial of weekly paclitaxel in patients with previously treated advanced urothelial cancer. *J Clin Oncol.* 2002;20:937–940.

20. McCaffrey JA, Hilton S, Mazumdar M, et al. Phase II trial of docetaxel in patients with advanced or metastatic transitional-cell carcinoma. *J Clin Oncol.* 1997;15:1853–1857.

21. Witte RS, Elson P, Bono B, et al. Eastern Cooperative Oncology Group phase II trial of ifosfamide in the treatment of previously treated advanced urothelial carcinoma. *J Clin Oncol.* 1997;15:589–593.

22. Lorusso V, Pollera CF, Antimi M, et al. A phase II study of gemcitabine in patients with transitional cell carcinoma of the urinary tract previously treated with platinum. Italian Co-operative Group on Bladder Cancer. *Eur J Cancer.* 1998;34:1208–1212.

23. Vaishampayan UN, Faulkner JR, Small EJ, et al. Phase II trial of carboplatin and paclitaxel in cisplatin-pretreated advanced transitional cell carcinoma: a Southwest Oncology Group study. *Cancer.* 2005;104:1627–1632.

24. Culine S, Theodore C, De Santis M, et al. A phase II study of vinflunine in bladder cancer patients progressing after first-line platinum-containing regimen. *Br J Cancer.* 2006;94:1395–1401.

25. Galsky MD, Mironov S, Iasonos A, et al. Phase II trial of pemetrexed as second-line therapy in patients with metastatic urothelial carcinoma. *Invest New Drugs.* 2007;25(3):265–270.

26.   Sweeney CJ, Roth BJ, Kabbinavar FF, et al. Phase II study of pemetrexed for second-line treatment of transitional cell cancer of the urothelium. *J Clin Oncol.* 2006;24:3451–3457.

27.   Bellmunt J, Theodore C, Demkov T, et al. Phase III trial of vinflunine plus best supportive care compared with best supportive care alone after a platinum-containing regimen in patients with advanced transitional cell carcinoma of the urothelial tract. *J Clin Oncol.* 2009;27:4454–4461.

28.   Hussain M, Vaishampayan U, Du W, et al. Combination paclitaxel, carboplatin, and gemcitabine is an active treatment for advanced urothelial cancer. *J Clin Oncol.* 2001; 19:2527–2533.

29.   Phillips G, Sanford B, Halabi S, et al. Phase II study of cisplatin (C), gemcitabine (G) and gefitinib for advanced urothelial carcinoma (UC): analysis of the second cohort of CALGB 90102. *J Clin Oncol.* 2006;24:Abstract 4578.

30.   Bellmunt J, Maroto P, Mellado B, et al. Phase II study of sunitinib as first line treatment in patients with advanced urothelial cancer ineligible for cisplatin-based chemotherapy. ASCO Genitourinary Oncology Symposium 2008: Abstract 291.

31.   Gallagher DJ, Milowsky MI, Gerst SR, et al. Phase II study of sunitinib in patients with metastatic urothelial cancer. *J Clin Oncol.* 2010;28:1373–1379.

32.   Galsky MD, Sonpavde G, Hellerstedt BA, et al. Phase II study of gemcitabine, cisplatin, and sunitinib in patients with advanced urothelial carcinoma. ASCO Genitourinary Oncology Symposium 2010:Abstract 276.

33.   Hahn NM, Stadler WM, Zon RT, et al. A multicenter phase II study of cisplatin (C), gemcitabine (G), and bevacizumab (B) as first-line chemotherapy for metastatic urothelial carcinoma (UC): Hoosier Oncology Group GU-0475. *J Clin Oncol.* 2009;27:Abstract 5018.

34.   Bajorin DF, Dodd PM, Mazumdar M, et al. Long-term survival in metastatic transitional-cell carcinoma and prognostic factors predicting outcome of therapy. *J Clin Oncol.* 1999;17:3173–3181.

35.   Dodd PM, McCaffrey JA, Herr H, et al. Outcome of post-chemotherapy surgery after treatment with methotrexate, vinblastine, doxorubicin, and cisplatin in patients with unresectable or metastatic transitional cell carcinoma. *J Clin Oncol.* 1999;17:2546–2552.

Nontransitional Cell Carcinomas of the Urothelial Tract

■ Overview

▣ Over 90% of cancers of the urothelial tract in the United States are transitional cell carcinomas.

▣ Mixed tumors, consisting of transitional cell carcinoma mixed with other elements (e.g., squamous cell carcinoma) are frequently encountered and generally considered a subset of transitional cell carcinomas.

▣ Nontransitional cell carcinomas include:
  • Epithelial subtypes
  • Squamous cell carcinoma
  • Adenocarcinomas
  • Small cell (neuroendocrine) carcinomas

▣ Nonepithelial subtypes
  • Sarcomas
  • Pheochromocytomas
  • Melanomas
  • Lymphomas

■ Squamous Cell Carcinomas

▣ Squamous cell carcinoma accounts for approximately 3–5% of bladder cancers in the United States but for 75% of bladder cancers in regions where schistosomiasis is endemic.

▣ Nonbilharzial squamous cell carcinoma of the bladder (squamous cell carcinoma not associated with schistosomiasis)
  • Surgery is the mainstay of treatment for squamous cell carcinoma of the bladder.

- Prognosis is generally poor, with a 5-year survival rate of approximately 35–50%. Local relapse and progression are particularly troublesome, with distant metastases occurring less frequently.
- The benefit of adjuvant radiation therapy and chemotherapy is unknown because randomized trials are not available in this rare patient population. Retrospective trials have suggested a possible benefit with the use of radiation therapy.[1]
- Squamous cell carcinomas of the bladder are generally thought to be chemotherapy-resistant tumors. However, a small prospective trial evaluating a regimen of ifosfamide, paclitaxel, and cisplatin in patients with advanced/metastatic nontransitional cell carcinomas of the urothelial tract did demonstrate a small proportion of objective responses.[2]

- Bilharzial squamous cell carcinoma of the bladder
  - Infection with the parasitic trematode *Schistosomia haematobium* is most prevalent in East Africa and the Middle East. This results in urinary tract disease known as bilharzial bladder disease. Bilharzial bladder disease is linked to the development of invasive carcinoma of the bladder. Approximately 75% of cases are squamous cell carcinomas, 20% are transitional cell carcinomas, and 5% are adenocarcinomas.
  - Radical cystectomy and lymph node dissection is the treatment of choice for localized bilharzial squamous cell carcinoma of the bladder.
  - An improvement in disease-free survival with the use of adjuvant radiation therapy has been demonstrated in a randomized trial of patients with pT3–T4 bilharzial squamous cell carcinoma of the bladder.[3]
  - Small randomized trials of neoadjuvant or adjuvant chemotherapy have also suggested an improvement in disease-free survival.[4]

■ Adenocarcinomas

- Primary adenocarcinomas of the bladder are the second most common nontransitional cell cancer arising in the urothelial tract in the United States and account for approximately 2% of bladder cancers overall in the United States.

■ Urachal adenocarcinomas

- A subset of adenocarcinomas of the bladder (approximately 10%) arise from the urachal remnant.[5]
- The diagnosis of urachal adenocarcinoma is suggested by the following:
  - Adenocarcinoma involving the dome of the bladder
  - Presence of a patent urachus
  - Absence of cystitis glandularis
  - No involvement or secondary involvement of the urothelium
- Surgical resection is the treatment of choice for localized urachal adenocarcinomas, and partial cystectomy (including en bloc resection of the bladder dome, urachal ligament, and umbilicus) is the recommended procedure. If the tumor cannot be resected with adequate margins, then a radical cystectomy should be performed.
- There is currently no proven role for adjuvant radiation or chemotherapy in patients with urachal adenocarcinoma. For patients with metastatic disease, regimens including 5-fluorouracil and/or cisplatin have shown some activity.[2,6,7]

■ Nonurachal adenocarcinomas of the bladder

- Radical cystectomy is the treatment of choice for the management of nonurachal adenocarcinomas of the bladder.
- There is currently no proven role for adjuvant radiation or chemotherapy.
- For patients with metastatic disease, the data to support the use of systemic chemotherapy are largely limited to case reports and small series.[2,8]

■ Small Cell Carcinomas

■ Small cell carcinomas of the bladder account for approximately 1% of bladder tumors in the United States.

■ For patients with no radiographic evidence of distant metastases, combined modality therapy is typically utilized based largely on retrospective series. Unlike the management of small cell lung cancer, surgery commonly plays a role, with many referral centers employing neoadjuvant chemotherapy with cisplatin-based chemotherapy followed by cystectomy.[9]

- A prospective phase II study exploring neoadjuvant chemotherapy followed by radical cystectomy in patients with small cell carcinoma of the bladder has been reported. In this trial, 18 patients with localized disease received alternating doublet chemotherapy with doxorubicin plus ifosfamide and cisplatin plus etoposide for four cycles, followed by surgery, and achieved a 5-year survival rate of 48%.[10]

- Regimens with activity in the treatment of extensive stage small cell lung cancer (e.g., etoposide plus carboplatin) are commonly utilized for the treatment of metastatic small cell carcinoma of the bladder.

■ References

1. Swanson DA, Liles A, Zagars GK. Preoperative irradiation and radical cystectomy for stages T2 and T3 squamous cell carcinoma of the bladder. *J Urol.* 1990;143:37–40.

2. Galsky MD, Iasonos A, Mironov S, et al. Prospective trial of ifosfamide, paclitaxel, and cisplatin in patients with advanced non-transitional cell carcinoma of the urothelial tract. *Urology.* 2007;69:255–259.

3. Zaghloul MS, Awwad HK, Akoush HH, et al. Postoperative radiotherapy of carcinoma in bilharzial bladder: improved disease free survival through improving local control. *Int J Radiat Oncol Biol Phys.* 1992;23:511–517.

4. Gad el Mawla N, Mansour MA, Eissa S, et al. A randomized pilot study of high-dose epirubicin as neoadjuvant chemotherapy in the treatment of cancer of the bilharzial bladder. *Ann Oncol.* 1991;2:137–140.

5. Manunta A, Vincendeau S, Kiriakou G, et al. Non-transitional cell bladder carcinomas. *BJU Int.* 2005;95:497–502.

6. Siefker-Radtke A. Urachal carcinoma: surgical and chemotherapeutic options. *Expert Rev Anticancer Ther.* 2006;6: 1715–1721.

7. Siefker-Radtke AO, Gee J, Shen Y, et al. Multimodality management of urachal carcinoma: the M. D. Anderson Cancer Center experience. *J Urol.* 2003;169:1295–1298.

8. Logothetis CJ, Samuels ML, Ogden S. Chemotherapy for adenocarcinomas of bladder and urachal origin: 5-fluorouracil, doxorubicin, and mitomycin-C. *Urology.* 1985;26:252–255.

9. Siefker-Radtke AO, Dinney CP, Abrahams NA, et al. Evidence supporting preoperative chemotherapy for small cell carcinoma of the bladder: a retrospective review of the M. D. Anderson cancer experience. *J Urol.* 2004;172: 481–484.

10. Siefker-Radtke A, Kamat AM, Grossman HB, et al. Final results from a phase II trial of systemic chemotherapy in a small cell urothelial cancer: evidence supporting neoadjuvant chemotherapy from the M. D. Anderson Cancer Center. *Proc Am Soc Clin Oncol.* 2007;25:Abstract 5083.

Cancers of
the Kidney

Renal Carcinoma: Epidemiology and Risk Factors

■ Epidemiology

- Each year in the United States, approximately 51,000 patients are diagnosed with renal carcinoma, and approximately 13,000 patients will succumb to their illness.[1]
- The incidence of renal carcinoma has increased over the past 20 years. This has been attributed to, at least in part, an increased incidence of incidentally detected tumors due to the widespread use of CT scanning.[2]
- Approximately 50% of patients with renal carcinoma present with, or develop, metastatic disease.

■ Demographics

- Renal carcinoma is most commonly diagnosed in patients 50–70 years old.
- Renal carcinoma is more common in men than women, with a ratio of approximately 2:1.

■ Risk Factors

- Cigarette smoking increases the risk of developing renal carcinoma approximately twofold. Smoking cessation is associated with a reduction in the relative risk compared with those people who continue to smoke.[3]
- Exposure to toxins, including cadmium, asbestos, and petroleum by-products, has been linked to a higher incidence of renal carcinoma.[4]
- Obesity and hypertension have been associated with an increased risk of developing renal carcinoma.[5]

- End-stage renal disease with acquired cystic kidney disease, particularly in patients on dialysis, is associated with an increased risk of developing renal carcinoma, approximately 20 times that of the general population.[6]

■ Genetic Disorders Associated with Renal Carcinoma

- Von Hippel–Lindau disease[7]
  - Autosomal dominant
  - Associated with abnormalities of chromosome 3p, leading to von Hippel–Lindau (VHL) gene mutations
  - Associated with the development of benign and malignant tumors of multiple organ systems, including:
    - Retinal angiomas
    - Cerebellar and spinal hemangioblastomas
    - Renal cell carcinomas
  - Typically multicentric and often bilateral renal carcinoma
  - Predominantly associated with clear cell (conventional type) renal carcinoma
- Birt-Hogg-Dube syndrome[8]
  - Autosomal dominant
  - Associated with abnormalities of chromosome 17p
  - Characterized by:
    - Prominent skin lesions (including fibrofolliculomas or hamartomas of the hair follicle)
    - Spontaneous pneumothoraces associated with lung cysts
    - Kidney cancers, particularly oncocytomas and chromophobe
- Hereditary papillary renal carcinoma[9]
  - Associated with abnormalities of the c-met oncogene on chromosome 7
  - Characterized by multiple, bilateral, papillary renal tumors
    - Reed syndrome (hereditary leiomyoma and renal cell cancer syndrome)[10]
  - Autosomal dominant

- Associated with mutations in the fumarate hydratase gene on chromosome 1
- Characterized by:
  - Cutaneous leiomyomas
  - Uterine fibroids
  - Renal carcinomas

■ References

1. Jemal A, Siegel R, Ward E, et al. Cancer statistics, 2007. *CA Cancer J Clin.* 2007;57:43–66.
2. Chow WH, Devesa SS, Warren JL, et al. Rising incidence of renal cell cancer in the United States. *JAMA.* 1999; 281:1628–1631.
3. Hunt JD, van der Hel OL, McMillan GP, et al. Renal cell carcinoma in relation to cigarette smoking: meta-analysis of 24 studies. *Int J Cancer.* 2005;114:101–108.
4. Mandel JS, McLaughlin JK, Schlehofer B, et al. International renal-cell cancer study. IV. Occupation. *Int J Cancer.* 1995;61:601–605.
5. Chow WH, Gridley G, Fraumeni JF Jr., et al. Obesity, hypertension, and the risk of kidney cancer in men. *N Engl J Med.* 2000;343:1305–1311.
6. Truong LD, Krishnan B, Cao JT, et al. Renal neoplasm in acquired cystic kidney disease. *Am J Kidney Dis.* 1995;26: 1–12.
7. Kim WY, Kaelin WG. Role of VHL gene mutation in human cancer. *J Clin Oncol.* 2004;22:4991–5004.
8. Pavlovich CP, Grubb RL 3rd, Hurley K, et al. Evaluation and management of renal tumors in the Birt-Hogg-Dube syndrome. *J Urol.* 2005;173:1482–1486.
9. Zbar B, Tory K, Merino M, et al. Hereditary papillary renal cell carcinoma. *J Urol.* 1994;151:561–566.
10. Refae MA, Wong N, Patenaude F, et al. Hereditary leiomyomatosis and renal cell cancer: an unusual and aggressive form of hereditary renal carcinoma. *Nat Clin Pract Oncol.* 2007; 4:256–261.

Renal Carcinoma: Diagnosis, Pathology, Pathogenesis, and Staging

■ Symptoms

▪ Hematuria, flank pain, and a palpable abdominal mass were historically the most common presenting symptoms/ signs of renal carcinoma. With the widespread use of CT scanning, a large proportion of renal carcinomas are detected incidentally, and few patients present with this classic triad.

▪ Scrotal varicoceles, particularly left sided, may be indicative of an underlying renal carcinoma that has obstructed the gonadal vein.

▪ Pain and weight loss are typically harbingers of advanced disease.

▪ Several paraneoplastic syndromes are associated with renal carcinoma, including:
  • Stauffer syndrome (hepatic dysfunction in the absence of liver metastases)
  • Fever
  • Hypercalcemia
  • Anemia
  • Erythrocytosis (secondary to production of erythropoietin)
  • Secondary amyloidosis

■ Initial Diagnostic Workup

▪ A CT scan or ultrasound of the abdomen are typically the initial studies that detect the presence of a renal neoplasm.

- Further evaluation of cystic renal masses depends on the presence of radiographic characteristics suggestive of a simple cyst versus a complex cyst. Simple cysts by ultrasound criteria require no further evaluation. If the cyst is questionable on ultrasound, a CT scan is generally performed, with further management necessary unless a simple cyst is confirmed (e.g., clearly delineated wall, lack of enhancement of intravenous contrast, water density).

- Solid renal masses are generally resected with a nephrectomy or partial nephrectomy given the likelihood of a renal neoplasm. Unlike most other areas of solid tumor oncology, a biopsy is generally not pursued prior to definitive surgery given the characteristic findings on imaging, concerns regarding sampling error, and concerns regarding tumor seeding. However, benign lesions remain in the differential diagnosis. In a series of patients undergoing nephrectomy for suspicious kidney lesions <7 cm in size, 16% of lesions were benign.[1] If metastatic disease is suspected, biopsy of a metastatic site is often the initial diagnostic procedure.

- The extent of local and regional involvement (perinephric invasion, renal vein invasion, regional lymphadenopathy, and invasion of adjacent organs) is generally assessed with a CT scan of the abdomen and pelvis.

- A CT scan of the chest (or chest x-ray) is performed to evaluate for the presence of pulmonary metastases.

- An MRI of the abdomen is performed if involvement of the inferior vena cava is suspected on CT scan.

- A bone scan and MRI of the brain are performed if there is clinical suspicion of metastases to these sites.

■ Pathology of Renal Carcinoma

- There are several histologic subtypes of renal carcinoma:
  - Clear cell (also known as conventional type)
    - Accounts for 70–85% of renal carcinomas.
    - Associated with chromosome 3p deletions and mutations of the von Hippel–Lindau gene (see Pathogenesis below).

- Papillary (also known as chromophilic)
  - Accounts for 10–15% of renal carcinomas.
  - Often multifocal and bilateral.
  - Inherited papillary renal carcinomas are associated with mutations of the c-met oncogene.
- Chromophobe
  - Accounts for 5–10% of renal carcinomas.
  - Associated with a favorable prognosis.
- Oncocytoma
  - Uncommon.
  - Rarely invasive and rarely metastasizes.
- Collecting duct (also known as Bellini tumor)
  - Uncommon.
  - Behave aggressively, and diagnosis is made at younger ages.
  - May be more closely related to transitional cell carcinomas than renal carcinomas at the molecular level.
- Renal medullary carcinoma
  - Uncommon.
  - Found almost exclusively in African Americans and is associated with sickle cell trait or sickle cell disease.
  - Behaves aggressively, with the majority of patients presenting with distant metastases.
- Wilms tumor
  - Most common malignant neoplasm of the urinary tract in children.
  - Peak incidence between the ages of 3 and 4 years.

■ Pathogenesis of Clear Cell Renal Carcinomas

- Clear cell renal carcinoma is characterized by frequent loss of the von Hippel–Lindau (VHL) tumor suppressor gene through deletion or posttranslational modification.[2]
- Functional *VHL* encodes a protein that targets hypoxia inducible factor (HIF) for degradation. As a result, inactivation of *VHL* leads to up-regulation of HIF. HIF leads to transcription of multiple genes involved in tumorigenesis, including vascular endothelial growth factor

(VEGF). Increased expression of VEGF results in tumor angiogenesis.[2]

■ Staging of Renal Carcinoma

- The TNM staging of renal carcinoma is detailed in **Tables 9.1** and **9.2**.

Table 9.1   TNM Staging in Renal Carcinoma

T Stage (Primary Tumor)	
T1	T1a—Tumor ≤4 cm in greatest dimension and limited to kidney
	T1b—Tumor >4 cm but <7 cm, and limited to kidney
T2	Tumor >7 cm in greatest dimension limited to the kidney
T3	T3a—Tumor directly invades the adrenal gland or perinephric tissues but not beyond Gerota's fascia
	T3b—Tumor grossly extends into the renal vein or its segmental (muscle-containing) branches, or vena cava below the diaphragm
	T3c—Tumor grossly extends into the vena cava above the diaphragm or invades the wall of the vena cava
T4	Tumor invades beyond Gerota's fascia
N Stage (Lymph Nodes)	
N0	No regional lymph node metastases are detected
N1	Metastasis in a single regional lymph node
N2	Metastases in more than one regional lymph node
M Stage (Metastases)	
M0	No distant metastases
M1	Distant metastases

Source: Used with the permission of the American Joint Committee on Cancer (AJCC), Chicago, Illinois. The original source for this material is the *AJCC Cancer Staging Manual,* Seventh Edition (2010), published by Springer Science and Business Media LLC, www.springer.com.

Table 9.2   Renal Carcinoma Stage Groupings

Stage Grouping	T Stage	N Stage	M Stage
I	T1	N0	M0
II	T2	N0	M0
III	T1 or T2	M0	
	T3	N0 or N1	M0
IV	T4	Any N	M0
	Any T	N2	M0
	Any T	Any N	M1

Source: Used with the permission of the American Joint Committee on Cancer (AJCC), Chicago, Illinois. The original source for this material is the *AJCC Cancer Staging Manual,* Seventh Edition (2010), published by Springer Science and Business Media LLC, www.springer.com.

■ References

1.   Snyder ME, Bach A, Kattan MW, et al. Incidence of benign lesions for clinically localized renal masses smaller than 7 cm in radiological diameter: influence of sex. *J Urol.* 2006;176: 2391–2395; discussion 2395–2396.
2.   Kim WY, Kaelin WG. Role of VHL gene mutation in human cancer. *J Clin Oncol.* 2004;22:4991–5004.

CHAPTER 10

Localized Renal Carcinoma

■ Management of Solid Renal Masses

■ As discussed in Chapter 9, solid renal masses are generally managed with surgery (e.g., nephrectomy, partial nephrectomy) as both a diagnostic and therapeutic maneuver, given the likelihood of a renal neoplasm based on imaging characteristics and concerns about inaccuracies and potential morbidity with percutaneous biopsies.

■ With the increased use of cross-sectional imaging, an increased number of small incidental solid renal masses are being identified.

■ In an analysis of small solid renal masses (mean lesion size at presentation 2.6 cm) that were observed for at least 1 year, the mean growth rate of these tumors was 0.28 cm/year (0.4 cm/year in tumors with pathologic confirmation of renal carcinoma).[1] The progression to metastatic disease was only 1% (3 of 286). However, baseline factors were insufficient to predict the natural history, and finding appropriate candidates for a surveillance approach remains a clinical dilemma.

■ In patients who are not surgical candidates, surveillance or ablative techniques (e.g., cryotherapy, radiofrequency ablation) can be considered.

■ The optimal approach for very small lesions (<1.5 cm) remains unclear. These lesions are often too small for adequate radiographic characterization, and follow-up is necessary.

■ Surgery for Renal Carcinoma

■ Radical nephrectomy involves ligation of the renal artery and vein and removal of the kidney, Gerota fascia, and ipsilateral adrenal gland.

- The operative mortality rate from a radical nephrectomy is approximately 2%. Complications include injury to the gastrointestinal organs or major blood vessels and secondary hemorrhage from the renal pedicle. Additional complications include ileus, wound infections, renal failure, myocardial infarction, congestive heart failure, thromboembolic disease, cerebrovascular accidents, and pneumonia.
- Although randomized comparisons have not been performed, large single and multi-institutional series have demonstrated that laparoscopic nephrectomy may be performed for tumors <10 cm without apparent compromise of oncologic outcomes.[2,3]
- The role of routine lymphadenectomy in patients with no evidence of preoperative lymph node involvement on cross-sectional imaging is controversial.
- Involvement of the inferior vena cava is not a contraindication to potentially curative surgery and can often be managed with nephrectomy and thrombectomy.
- Nephron-sparing approaches
  - Renal insufficiency is a potential long-term complication of nephrectomy. In a retrospective analysis from a single institution, 12% of patients had a creatinine level of ≥2.0 mg/dL at a median follow-up of 21 months from surgery.[4]
  - Several approaches to spare renal function have been explored, including partial nephrectomy and ablative procedures.
  - Outcomes with partial nephrectomy for small tumors appear similar to outcomes with radical nephrectomy.
  - Cryoablation and radiofrequency ablation are procedures that can be performed with a percutaneous approach. These procedures are attractive for patients who are not surgical candidates or for patients with multifocal tumors. However, with these approaches, the diagnosis of malignancy may be limited to fine-needle aspirate biopsy material or might not be confirmed at all.

■ Prognosis After Surgery for Renal Carcinoma

- ▨ Although TNM stage groupings define subsets of patients with renal cell carcinoma (RCC) with different outcomes, several analyses have been conducted in an attempt to refine prognosis in patients undergoing radical nephrectomy.

- ▨ Investigators at the University of California–Los Angeles (UCLA) performed a study of 661 patients with either localized or metastatic RCC who had undergone nephrectomy.[5] Multiple factors were evaluated for their impact on survival. The final model, coined the UCLA Integrated Staging System (UISS), consisted of TNM stage, nuclear grade, and performance status. This system predicted survival better than TNM stage alone, allowing patients to be classified into five different risk groups with distinct outcomes (see **Table 10.1**). The model has been externally validated using several large data sets.[6,7]

Table 10.1   Prognosis After Radical Nephrectomy Based on the UCLA Integrated Staging System (UISS)

UISS Stage	TNM Stage	Fuhrman Grade	PS	5-year Survival Rate
I	I	1 or 2	0	94%
II	I	1 or 2	1 or more	67%
	I	3 or 4	Any	
	II	Any	Any	
	III	Any	0	
	III	1	1 or more	
III	III	2–4	1 or more	39%
	IV	1 or 2	0	
IV	IV	3 or 4	0	23%
	IV	1–3	1 or more	
V	IV	4	1 or more	0

TNM, Tumor-node-metastases staging system; PS, performance status.

Source: Adapted from Zisman et al.[5]

- Investigators at Memorial Sloan-Kettering have developed a points-based nomogram to individualize predictions regarding prognosis in patients with renal carcinoma postnephrectomy based on several clinical variables that include patient symptoms, tumor histology, tumor size, and pathologic stage. This nomogram is available at www.nomograms.org.

■ Adjuvant Therapy for Renal Carcinoma Postnephrectomy

- Based on the activity of immunotherapy in patients with metastatic RCC, several randomized trials explored the use of immunotherapy in the adjuvant setting after nephrectomy for RCC (see **Table 10.2**). These trials differed slightly in the immunotherapy regimens employed.

Table 10.2   Trials of Adjuvant Immunotherapy in Renal Carcinoma

Reference	n	Eligibility	Treatment Arms	Survival Benefit?
Porzsolt et al.[8]	283	T3b–4 or N1–N3	IFNa vs. observation	No
Pizzocaro et al.[9]	270	Robson stage II or III	IFNa–2a vs. observation	No
Atzpodien et al.[10]	247	Robson stage II or III	IFNa–2a vs. observation	No
Clark et al.[11]	203	Stage III*	IFNa plus 5-FU vs. low-dose SC IL-2 vs. observation	No
Passalacqua et al.[12]	69	T3b–4 or N1–3 or resected M1	High-dose IL-2 vs. observation	No
Fyfe et al.[13]	310	T2–T3c and/or N0–N3	SC IL-2 + SC IFN vs. observation	No

IFN, interferon; IL, interleukin; 5-FU, 5-fluorouracil; SC, subcutaneous.

*Stage III or completely resected local recurrence or solitary metastasis.

Nonetheless, these trials all failed to demonstrate a survival benefit with the use of immunotherapy; the current standard of care remains surveillance in the absence of an available clinical trial.

▪ Tumor vaccines have also been evaluated as adjuvant therapy in patients postnephrectomy for RCC in phase III trials without a demonstrable survival benefit.[14]

▪ Several large phase III clinical trials are currently exploring the role of novel multitargeted tyrosine kinase inhibitors as adjuvant therapy postnephrectomy for RCC.

▪ References

1. Chawla SN, Crispen PL, Hanlon AL, et al. The natural history of observed enhancing renal masses: meta-analysis and review of the world literature. *J Urol.* 2006;175:425–431.

2. Dunn MD, Portis AJ, Shalhav AL, et al. Laparoscopic versus open radical nephrectomy: a 9-year experience. *J Urol.* 2000;164:1153–1159.

3. Gill IS, Meraney AM, Schweizer DK, et al. Laparoscopic radical nephrectomy in 100 patients: a single center experience from the United States. *Cancer.* 2001;92:1843–1855.

4. Sorbellini M, Kattan MW, Snyder ME, et al. Prognostic nomogram for renal insufficiency after radical or partial nephrectomy. *J Urol.* 2006;176:472–476; discussion 476.

5. Zisman A, Pantuck AJ, Dorey F, et al. Improved prognostication of renal cell carcinoma using an integrated staging system. *J Clin Oncol.* 2001;19:1649–1657.

6. Han KR, Bleumer I, Pantuck AJ, et al. Validation of an integrated staging system toward improved prognostication of patients with localized renal cell carcinoma in an international population. *J Urol.* 2003;170:2221–2224.

7. Patard JJ, Kim HL, Lam JS, et al. Use of the University of California Los Angeles integrated staging system to predict survival in renal cell carcinoma: an international multicenter study. *J Clin Oncol.* 2004;22:3316–3322.

8. Porzsolt F. Adjuvant therapy of renal cell cancer with interferon alfa-2a. *Proc Am Soc Clin Oncol.* 1992;11:Absract 622.

9. Pizzocaro G, Piva L, Colavita M, et al. Interferon adjuvant to radical nephrectomy in Robson stages II and III renal cell carcinoma: a multicentric randomized study. *J Clin Oncol.* 2001;19:425–431.

10. Atzpodien J, Schmitt E, Gertenbach U, et al. Adjuvant treatment with interleukin-2- and interferon-alpha2a-based chemoimmunotherapy in renal cell carcinoma post tumour

nephrectomy: results of a prospectively randomised trial of the German Cooperative Renal Carcinoma Chemoimmuno-therapy Group (DGCIN). *Br J Cancer.* 2005;92:843–846.

11. Clark JI, Atkins MB, Urba WJ, et al. Adjuvant high-dose bolus interleukin-2 for patients with high-risk renal cell carcinoma: a Cytokine Working Group randomized trial. *J Clin Oncol.* 2003;21:3133–3140.

12. Passalacqua R, Buzio C, Buti S, et al. Adjuvant low-dose interleukin-2 plus interferone-alpha in operable renal cell cancer. A phase III, randomized, multicenter, independent trial of the Italian Oncology Group for Clinical Research. *Proc Am Soc Clin Oncol.* 2007;25:Abstract 5028.

13. Fyfe G, Fisher RI, Rosenberg SA, et al. Results of treatment of 255 patients with metastatic renal cell carcinoma who received high-dose recombinant interleukin-2 therapy. *J Clin Oncol.* 1995;13:688–696.

14. Jocham D, Richter A, Hoffmann L, et al. Adjuvant autologous renal tumour cell vaccine and risk of tumour progression in patients with renal-cell carcinoma after radical nephrectomy: phase III, randomised controlled trial. *Lancet.* 2004;363: 594–599.

Metastatic Renal Carcinoma

■ Immunotherapy for Renal Carcinoma

▪ A small minority of patients with metastatic RCC develop spontaneous regression of disease. For example, in a randomized trial of interferon versus placebo, the overall response rate on the placebo arm was 6.6%, with durable complete responses in 1% of patients. The host immune system is felt to be responsible for these spontaneous regressions, and several approaches have been explored in an attempt to stimulate the immune system as therapy for metastatic RCC.

▪ High-dose interleukin-2 (IL-2)

  • Multiple phase II studies have explored high-dose bolus IL-2 for treatment of metastatic RCC.

  • Treatment generally consisted of 15-minute intravenous infusions of IL-2 every 8 hours for up to 14 consecutive doses over 5 days, as tolerated. A second identical cycle of treatment was scheduled following 5 to 9 days of rest, and courses could be repeated every 6 to 12 weeks in stable or responding patients.

  • In a cohort of 255 patients treated in seven phase II trials, the overall response rate was 14% (90% CI 10–19%), with 12 (5%) complete responses and 24 (9%) partial responses. Responses occurred in all sites of disease.[1]

  • Treatment with high-dose IL-2 was associated with severe acute toxicities, including hypotension, cardiac arrhythmias, fever/chills, nausea/vomiting, renal failure, peripheral edema, and neurotoxicity. In the cohort of 255 patients, 4% died due to adverse events.

  • With extended follow-up, the median duration for all complete responses had not been reached, but was at least 80 months (range, 7–131 months). These data suggest a small subset of patients with metastatic RCC can be cured with high-dose IL-2.[2] U.S. Food and Drug Administration (FDA) approval of IL-2 for treatment of metastatic RCC was based on the durable complete responses in this subset of patients.

- High-dose IL-2 is administered in select centers with experience managing the severe acute toxicities associated with treatment.

- Given the potential for durable complete responses in a small subset of patients, high-dose IL-2 is considered a standard first-line treatment approach for patients with a good performance status and adequate organ function. Efforts to more appropriately select patients who are likely to respond to high-dose IL-2 have included analyses of both clinical and molecular factors. The following have been associated with an increased likelihood of response to high-dose IL-2:
  - Prior nephrectomy
  - Time from nephrectomy to treatment of at least 1 year
  - Good performance status
  - Absence of bone or liver metastases
  - Clear cell (conventional type) histology
  - High level of expression of carbonic anhydrase IX

- Interferon alfa
  - Several trials have demonstrated the activity of interferon alfa in the treatment of metastatic RCC.
  - In a trial comparing continuous infusion IL-2, subcutaneous interferon alfa-2a, or the combination thereof, the response rates were 6.5%, 7.5%, and 18.6%, respectively.[3] However, there was no difference in overall survival among the arms.
  - Trials comparing interferon plus vinblastine versus vinblastine alone versus megesterol have suggested a survival benefit with the use of interferon in metastatic RCC.[4,5] A Cochrane review of immunotherapy in RCC reported an average improvement in median survival of 2.6 months with interferon versus a variety of comparative regimens.[6]

- Side effects associated with interferon include flulike symptoms, depression, myelosuppression, and liver function test abnormalities.
- Interferon-alfa is associated with a similar overall response rate to high-dose IL-2. However, most of the responses are partial and short-lived, and evidence of durable complete responses as observed in a subset of patients treated with high-dose IL-2 is lacking. Given the ease of administration (subcutaneous) and favorable side effect profile, interferon alfa was the most commonly employed first-line treatment for metastatic RCC prior to the advent of the multitargeted tyrosine kinase inhibitors and mammalian target of rapamycin (mTOR) inhibitors (see below).

■ Targeted Therapies for Renal Carcinoma

- Clear cell renal carcinoma is characterized by frequent loss of the von Hippel–Lindau (VHL) tumor suppressor gene and subsequent up-regulation of HIF-1-α. The latter results in transcription of several genes central to tumorigenesis, including vascular endothelial growth factor (VEGF), platelet-derived growth factor (PDGF), and fibroblast growth factor (FGF). Therefore, there is a clear rationale for targeting these growth factor pathways in metastatic RCC.
- Bevacizumab
  - Bevacizumab is a monoclonal antibody that binds and neutralizes VEGF.
  - In a trial that demonstrated "proof of concept" for targeting VEGF in RCC, 166 patients with metastatic RCC (refractory to IL-2) were randomized to bevacizumab at two different dose levels (10 mg/kg every 2 weeks or 3 mg/kg every 2 weeks) versus placebo (see **Table 11.1**).[7] Treatment with bevacizumab 10 mg/kg was associated with a prolongation of progression-free survival of 4.8 months, compared with 2.5 months with placebo.

Table 11.1   Randomized Trials of Novel Agents in Renal Carcinoma

Treatment Arms	Patient Population	Phase	n	Median PFS	Median OS
Sunitinib vs. IFN[8]	First-line Good/intermediate risk	III	750	11 vs. 5 months*	NA
Sorafenib vs. placebo[9]	Second-line Good/intermediate risk	III	905	24 vs. 12 weeks*	19.3 vs. 15.9 months*
Sorafenib vs. IFN[10]	First-line Good risk	II	189	5.7 vs. 5.6 months	NA
Lapatinib vs. hormones[11]	Second-line EGFR or Erb2 positive	III	417	15.3 vs. 15.4 weeks	46.9 vs. 43.1 weeks**
Bevacizumab vs. placebo[12]	Second-line	II	116	4.8 vs. 2.5 months*	NA
Bevacizumab + erlotinib vs. bevacizumab[13]	First-line	II	104	9.9 vs. 8.5 months	NA
Temsirolimus vs. IFN[14]	First-line Poor risk	III	626	3.7 vs. 1.9 months*	10.9 vs. 7.3 months*

Bevacizumab + IFN vs. bevacizumab + placebo[15]	First-line	III	649	10.2 vs. 5.4 *	NA
Becacizumab + IFN vs. IFN[1]	First-line	III	732	8.5 vs. 5.2 months	18.3 vs. 17.4 months
Everolimus vs. placebo[2]	Second-line	III	410	4.0 vs 1.9 months*	NA
Pazopanib vs. placebo[3]	First-line/Second-line	III	435	9.2 vs 4.2 months*	NA

PFS, progression-free survival; OS, overall survival; IFN, interferon; NA, not available; EGFR, epidermal growth factor receptor.

*Statistically significant.

**Statistically significant benefit for the subgroup of patients with 31 EGFR overexpression in favor of lapatinib.

[1]Rini B, Halabi S, Rosenberg JE, et al. Phase III trial of bevacizuman plus interferon alfa versus interferon alfa monotherapy in patients with metastatic renal cell carcinoma: final results of CALGB 90206. *J Clin Oncol.* 2010;13:2137–43.

[2]Motzer RJ, Escudier B, Oudard S, et al. Efficacy of everolimus in advanced renal cell carcinoma: a double-blind, randomised, placebo-controlled phase III trial. *Lancet.* 2008;9637:449–56.

[3]Sternberg CN, Davis ID, Mardiak J et al. Pazopanib in locally advanced or metastatic renal cell carcinoma: results of a randomized phase III trial. *J Clin Oncol.* 2010;28(6):1061–8.

- Two randomized phase III trials (CALGB-90206 and the European AVOREN study) have compared bevacizumab plus interferon versus bevacizumab plus placebo as first-line treatment in patients with metastatic RCC (see Table 11.1). The AVOREN study demonstrated a significant improvement in progression-free survival in the bevacizumab plus interferon arm (10.2 months versus 5.4 months, $p < 0.0001$).[15]
- Common side effects with bevacizumab include hypertension, proteinuria, and fatigue. Hemorrhage, gastrointestinal perforation, and thromboembolic disease were uncommon in the RCC studies.
- Bevacizumab in combination with interferon was approved by the U.S. FDA for the treatment of metastatic renal carcinoma in July 2009.
- Sunitinib
  - Sunitinib is an orally bioavailable potent inhibitor of multiple receptor tyrosine kinases, including VEGFR types 1 to 3 and PDGF.
  - Two phase II trials evaluated the activity of sunitinib in patients with disease progression despite prior treatment with cytokine therapy (interferon or interleukin).[16,17]
    - Sunitinib was administered at a dose of 50 mg PO daily for 4 weeks followed by a 2-week rest period.
    - A pooled analysis was performed on 168 patients. The objective response rate was 34% (95% CI 25–44%), with a median progression-free survival of 8.3 months.
    - Given the impressive level of activity in cytokine-refractory patients, based on these phase II trials, the U.S. FDA approved sunitinib for the treatment of RCC in January 2006.
    - The most common adverse events were fatigue, diarrhea, neutropenia, elevation of lipase levels, and anemia. Other toxicities observed with sunitinib include hand-foot syndrome (redness, swelling, and pain on the palms of the hands and/or the soles of the feet) and thyroid function abnormalities.
  - Given the promising results with sunitinib in cytokine-refractory patients, a large randomized phase III trial

compared sunitinib versus interferon in previously untreated patients (see Table 11.1).[8]

- The median progression-free survival was 11 months
  for the sunitinib arm and 5 months for the interferon arm (HR 0.415, $p < 0.000001$).
- Adverse events leading to withdrawal from the
  study occurred in 8% of patients on sunitinib and
  13% on interferon.
- Patients in the sunitinib group reported a significantly better quality of life.
- Based on these results, sunitinib has become a standard first-line treatment option for patients with
  metastatic RCC.

- Sorafenib
  - Sorafenib is an orally bioavailable potent inhibitor of
    Raf-kinase in addition to the receptor tyrosine kinases
    VEGFR2, PDGFR, Flt3, and c-KIT.
  - A large phase II randomized discontinuation trial eval-
    uated the activity of sorafenib 400 mg PO twice daily
    as second-line therapy for metastatic RCC. The ma-
    jority of patients had received prior cytokine therapy
    (see Table 11.1).[18]
    - The primary endpoint was progression-free survival
      at 24 weeks after the initiation of sorafenib.
    - Seventy-three patients had tumor shrinkage of >25%
      and continued sorafenib until disease progression.
    - Sixty-five patients with stable disease at 12 weeks
      were randomly assigned to sorafenib or placebo. At
      24 weeks, 50% of the sorafenib-treated patients were
      progression free versus 18% of the placebo-treated
      patients ($p = 0.0077$).
    - Common side effects with sorafenib included fatigue,
      hand-foot syndrome, diarrhea, and hypertension.
  - Based on the promising results of the randomized dis-
    continuation trial, a randomized phase III trial known
    as TARGET (Treatment Approaches in RCC Global
    Evaluation Trial) was performed (see Table 11.1).[9]
    - The TARGET trial enrolled 905 patients with met-
      astatic clear cell RCC who had progressed on one
      prior systemic therapy.

- Patients were randomized to sorafenib versus placebo, with overall survival as the primary endpoint.
- A planned interim analysis of progression-free survival demonstrated a statistically significant benefit of sorafenib over placebo. The median progression-free survival was 5.5 months in the sorafenib group and 2.8 months in the placebo group (HR = 0.44; 95% CI 0.35–0.55; $p < 0.01$). As a result, cross-over of patients on the placebo arm to treatment with sorafenib was permitted.

- Sorafenib was approved by the U.S. FDA for the treatment of advanced RCC in December 2005.
- Although no randomized phase III data are available exploring the efficacy of sorafenib as a first-line treatment for metastatic RCC, a randomized phase II trial of sorafenib versus interferon as first-line therapy has been completed (see Table 11.1).[10]
  - The primary endpoint was progression-free survival.
  - The median progression-free survival was 5.7 months (95% CI 5.0–7.4 months) versus 5.6 months (95% CI 3.7–7.4 months) for sorafenib versus interferon, respectively.

- Temsirolimus
  - Temsirolimus is an intravenously administered inhibitor of mTOR (mammalian target of rapamycin). Activated mTOR increases the expression of several proteins, including hypoxia inducible factor (HIF); notably, HIF expression is also up-regulated by inactivation of VHL. The result of HIF up-regulation is increased expression of several downstream growth factors, including VEGF. Inhibition of mTOR has been demonstrated to inhibit translation of HIF.
  - A randomized phase II study explored three different dose levels of weekly intravenous temsirolimus in patients with cytokine-refractory RCC.[19]
    - The objective response rate was 7%, with a median time to progression of 5.8 months and a median survival of 15 months.
    - When compared with historical controls, patients with poor-risk disease appeared to derive the most benefit from temsirolimus.

- ▨ Side effects with temsirolimus included rash, asthenia, mucositis, nausea, edema, and anorexia. The most common laboratory abnormalities included anemia, hyperglycemia, hyperlipidemia, hypertriglyceridemia, and liver function test abnormalities.
- A phase III study compared first-line treatment with temsirolimus versus interferon versus temsirolimus plus interferon in 626 patients with metastatic RCC and poor-risk features (see Table 11.1).[14]
  - ▨ Side effects more common in the temsirolimus arm included rash, peripheral edema, hyperglycemia, and hyperlipidemia. Asthenia was more common in the interferon arm. Notably, serious adverse events were more common in patients receiving interferon compared with temsirolimus.
  - ▨ The median survival was superior in the temsirolimus-alone arm compared with interferon alone (10.9 months versus 7.3 months, HR 0.73, $p <$ 0.007), while the combination arm was not superior to interferon alone (8.4 months, HR 0.95, $p = 0.69$). The combination arm was likely not superior due to a lower dose of temsirolimus used with the combination regimen.
  - ▨ Temsirolimus was approved by the U.S. FDA for the treatment of advanced RCC in May 2007.
- ▨ The first randomized phase III trial evaluating treatment for patients whose disease had progressed on sunitinib, sorafenib, or both compared the oral mTOR inhibitor everolimus versus placebo.[20]
  - There was a statistically significant improvement in median progression-free survival: 4.0 months (95% CI 3.7–5.5) in the everolimus arm versus 1.9 months (95% CI 1.8–1.9) in the placebo arm.
  - Stomatitis, rash, and fatigue were the most common side effects of everolimus.
  - Pneumonitis was detected in 22% of patients in the everolimus group.
  - Based on these results, everolimus was approved by the U.S. FDA for the treatment of renal carcinoma in March 2009.

Table 11.2   Proposed Treatment Algorithm for Advanced Renal Carcinoma in 2008

Line of Treatment	Patient Population	Treatment
First-line	Selected patients	High-dose IL-2
	Good/intermediate risk	Sunitinib
		Bevacizumab + IFN
		Pazopanib
	Poor risk	Temsirolimus
Second-line	Prior cytokines	Sunitinib or Pazopanib or Sorafenib
	Prior TKIs	Everolimus
	Prior m-TOR inhibitors	No standard therapy

TKIs, tyrosine kinase inhibitors; IFN, interferon; m-TOR, mammalian target of rapamycin; IL-2, interleukin-2.

- Based on the available data, a common algorithm for treatment selection for patients with metastatic renal carcinoma is outlined in **Table 11.2**.

■ Prognosis in Advanced Renal Carcinoma

- Several analyses have defined pretreatment variables associated with outcomes in patients with advanced renal carcinoma.
- The classification scheme developed by Motzer et al. is among the most widely used prognostic systems and has been externally validated (see **Table 11.3**).[21,22] Several analyses have explored prognostic factors in the age of targeted therapies and have confirmed and expanded on these prognostic factors.

■ Role of Surgery in Advanced Renal Carcinoma

- Nephrectomy
  - The role of cytoreductive nephrectomy or debulking nephrectomy in patients with metastatic disease has been explored in two randomized trials.
    - In a trial conducted by the Southwest Oncology Group (SWOG), 246 patients with metastatic

Table 11.3 Memorial Sloan-Kettering Risk Groups in Patients with Advanced Renal Carcinoma

Risk Group	Number of Risk Factors	Median Survival
Favorable	None	30 months
Intermediate	1–2	14 months
Poor	≥3	6 months

Risk factors include hemoglobin <10 mg/dL, lactate dehydrogenase >1.5 times upper limit of normal, corrected calcium >10 mg/dL, Karnofsky performance status <80%, and time interval from diagnosis to treatment of <1 year.

Source: Data derived from Motzer et al.[22]

renal carcinoma were randomized to treatment with interferon or treatment with radical nephrectomy followed by interferon.[23] The median survival was 11.1 months for patients assigned to the nephrectomy arm, compared with 8.1 months for patients treated with interferon alone ($p = 0.05$).

- ▦ A smaller trial with an identical design was conducted by the EORTC.[24] The median duration of survival favored patients undergoing radical nephrectomy (17 months versus 7 months, HR 0.54, 0.31–0.94).[24]
- The role of nephrectomy in patients treated with multi-targeted tyrosine kinase inhibitors or mTOR inhibitors is unclear. However, many of the trials that led to the approval of these agents did require patients to undergo nephrectomy prior to enrollment.
- Palliative nephrectomy for symptoms due to local progression (e.g., hematuria, pain) is also commonly performed.
- ▦ Metastasectomy
  - Several studies have reported prolonged survival with resection of metastatic sites in patients with renal carcinoma. The largest experience reported has been with resecting pulmonary metastases, with 5-year survival rates of 20–50%.[25]

• A retrospective series analyzed 152 resections of RCC metastases in 101 patients.[26] Resections were performed at several different locations, including lung, bone, and lymph nodes. The median survival from the time of metastasectomy was 28 months. Better survival was found for lung metastases compared with other locations and for patients without clinical evidence of disease after metastasectomy. A tumor-free interval of >2 years was associated with a longer disease-specific survival after metastasectomy. Long-term disease-free survival (>5 years) was observed in 7%.

■ References

1. Fyfe G, Fisher RI, Rosenberg SA, et al. Results of treatment of 255 patients with metastatic renal cell carcinoma who received high-dose recombinant interleukin-2 therapy. *J Clin Oncol.* 1995;13:688–696.

2. Fisher RI, Rosenberg SA, Fyfe G. Long-term survival update for high-dose recombinant interleukin-2 in patients with renal cell carcinoma. *Cancer J Sci Am.* 2000;6(suppl 1): S55–S57.

3. Negrier S, Escudier B, Lasset C, et al. Recombinant human interleukin-2, recombinant human interferon alfa-2a, or both in metastatic renal-cell carcinoma. Groupe Francais d'Immunotherapie. *N Engl J Med.* 1998;338:1272–1278.

4. Interferon-alpha and survival in metastatic renal carcinoma: early results of a randomised controlled trial. Medical Research Council Renal Cancer Collaborators. *Lancet.* 1999; 353:14–17.

5. Pyrhonen S, Salminen E, Ruutu M, et al. Prospective randomized trial of interferon alfa-2a plus vinblastine versus vinblastine alone in patients with advanced renal cell cancer. *J Clin Oncol.* 1999;17:2859–2867.

6. Coppin C, Porzsolt F, Awa A, et al. Immunotherapy for advanced renal cell cancer. *Cochrane Database Syst Rev.* 2005:CD001425.

7. Yang JC, Haworth L, Sherry RM, et al. A randomized trial of bevacizumab, an anti-vascular endothelial growth factor antibody, for metastatic renal cancer. *N Engl J Med.* 2003; 349:427–434.

8. Motzer RJ, Hutson TE, Tomczak P, et al. Sunitinib versus interferon alfa in metastatic renal-cell carcinoma. *N Engl J Med.* 2007;356:115–124.

9. Escudier B, Eisen T, Stadler WM, et al. Sorafenib in advanced clear-cell renal-cell carcinoma. *N Engl J Med.* 2007;356: 125–134.

10. Szczylik C, Demkow T, Staehler M, et al. Randomized phase II trial of first-line treatment with sorafenib versus interferon in patients with advanced renal cell carcinoma: final results. *Proc Am Soc Clin Oncol.* 2007;25:Abstract 5025.

11. Ravaud A, Gardner J, Hawkins R, et al. Efficacy of lapatinib in patients with high tumor EGFR expression: results of a phase III trial in advanced renal cell carcinoma. *Proc Am Soc Clin Oncol.* 2006;24:Abstract 4502.

12. Yang JC. Bevacizumab for patients with metastatic renal cancer: an update. *Clin Cancer Res.* 2004;10:6367S–6370S.

13. Bukowski RM, Kabbinavar FF, Figlin RA, et al. Randomized phase II study of erlotinib combined with bevacizumab compared with bevacizumab alone in metastatic renal cell cancer. *J Clin Oncol.* 2007;25:4536–4541.

14. Hudes G, Carducci M, Tomczak P, et al. Temsirolimus, interferon alfa, or both for advanced renal-cell carcinoma. *N Engl J Med.* 2007;356:2271–2281.

15. Escudier B, Pluzanska A, Koralewski P, et al. Bevacizumab plus interferon alfa-2a for treatment of metastatic renal cell carcinoma: a randomised, double-blind phase III trial. *Lancet.* 2007;370:2103–2111.

16. Motzer RJ, Michaelson MD, Redman BG, et al. Activity of SU11248, a multitargeted inhibitor of vascular endothelial growth factor receptor and platelet-derived growth factor receptor, in patients with metastatic renal cell carcinoma. *J Clin Oncol.* 2006;24:16–24.

17. Motzer RJ, Rini BI, Bukowski RM, et al. Sunitinib in patients with metastatic renal cell carcinoma. *JAMA.* 2006;295: 2516–2524.

18. Ratain MJ, Eisen T, Stadler WM, et al. Phase II placebo-controlled randomized discontinuation trial of sorafenib in patients with metastatic renal cell carcinoma. *J Clin Oncol.* 2006;24:2505–2512.

19. Atkins MB, Hidalgo M, Stadler WM, et al. Randomized phase II study of multiple dose levels of CCI-779, a novel mammalian target of rapamycin kinase inhibitor, in patients with advanced refractory renal cell carcinoma. *J Clin Oncol.* 2004;22:909–918.

20. Motzer RJ, Escudier B, Oudard S, et al. Efficacy of ever-olimus in advanced renal cell carcinoma: a double-blind, randomised, placebo-controlled phase III trial. *Lancet.* 2008; 372:449–456.

21. Mekhail TM, Abou-Jawde RM, Boumerhi G, et al. Validation and extension of the Memorial Sloan-Kettering prognos-tic factors model for survival in patients with previously

untreated metastatic renal cell carcinoma. *J Clin Oncol.* 2005;23:832–841.

22. Motzer RJ, Bacik J, Murphy BA, et al. Interferon-alfa as a comparative treatment for clinical trials of new therapies against advanced renal cell carcinoma. *J Clin Oncol.* 2002; 20:289–296.

23. Flanigan RC, Salmon SE, Blumenstein BA, et al. Nephrectomy followed by interferon alfa-2b compared with interferon alfa-2b alone for metastatic renal-cell cancer. *N Engl J Med.* 2001;345:1655–1659.

24. Mickisch GH, Garin A, van Poppel H, et al. Radical nephrectomy plus interferon-alfa-based immunotherapy compared with interferon alfa alone in metastatic renal-cell carcinoma: a randomised trial. *Lancet.* 2001;358:966–970.

25. Murthy SC, Kim K, Rice TW, et al. Can we predict long-term survival after pulmonary metastasectomy for renal cell carcinoma? *Ann Thorac Surg.* 2005;79:996–1003.

26. van der Poel HG, Roukema JA, Horenblas S, et al. Metastasectomy in renal cell carcinoma: a multicenter retrospective analysis. *Eur Urol.* 1999;35:197–203.

Cancers of
the Testis

Testicular Cancer: Epidemiology and Risk Factors

■ Epidemiology and Demographics

▪ Each year in the United States, approximately 8,000 patients are diagnosed with testicular germ cell tumors. However, fewer than 400 patients will succumb to their illness.[1]

▪ The 5-year survival rate for testicular germ cell tumors is over 95%.

▪ Several studies suggest that the incidence of testicular germ cell tumors is increasing. An analysis of the Connecticut Cancer Registry showed that the incidence of testis cancer had increased 3.5-fold over the past 60 years.[1]

▪ Testicular germ cell tumors are the most common solid tumors in men ages 15–35.

■ Risk Factors

▪ Intratubular germ cell neoplasia[2]
  • Premalignant condition is also known as carcinoma in situ.
  • Present in approximately 90% of orchiectomy specimens adjacent to testicular germ cell tumors.
  • Patients with intratubular germ cell neoplasia have an approximately 50% probability of progressing to frank germ-cell neoplasm within 5 years.
  • The optimal management of patients with intratubular germ cell neoplasia is not clear.
▪ Cryptorchidism (absent or undescended testicle)[3]
  • The incidence of testicular germ cell cancers in patients with cryptorchidism is approximately 1:1,000–2,500.

- Approximately 10% of testicular germ cell tumors occur in the setting of an undescended testicle.
- The germ cell tumor may occur in the descended or contralateral testicle.
- Orchiopexy does not eliminate the risk of developing a germ cell tumor but likely reduces the risk and also allows earlier detection.

▪ Second primary testicular germ cell tumor
- Approximately 2% of men undergoing an orchiectomy for a testicular germ cell tumor will develop a germ cell tumor in the contralateral testicle.

▪ Family history
▪ HIV infection
▪ Down syndrome
▪ Klinefelter syndrome
▪ Exposure to estrogens in utero

▪ References

1. Zheng T, Holford TR, Ma Z, et al. Continuing increase in incidence of germ-cell testis cancer in young adults: experience from Connecticut, USA, 1935–1992. *Int J Cancer.* 1996;65:723–729.

2. Dieckmann KP, Skakkebaek NE. Carcinoma in situ of the testis: review of biological and clinical features. *Int J Cancer.* 1999;83:815–822.

3. Abratt RP, Reddi VB, Sarembock LA. Testicular cancer and cryptorchidism. *Br J Urol.* 1992;70:656–659.

Testicular Cancer: Diagnosis, Pathology, and Staging

■ Symptoms

- Although a painless testicular mass is often described as the classic presentation for a testicular germ cell tumor, most men will report pain in the abdomen or scrotum.
- Gynecomastia and/or nipple tenderness may be present, particularly in the setting of elevated human chorionic gonadotropin.
- Back pain may be present in association with retroperitoneal lymphadenopathy.
- Other signs and symptoms may be associated with the presence or location of metastatic disease.

■ Initial Diagnostic Workup

- Solid testicular masses should be considered germ cell tumors until proven otherwise.
- A scrotal ultrasound is typically the initial imaging study utilized to evaluate a testicular mass. The ultrasound can both confirm the presence of a solid mass and detect the presence of findings characteristic of seminoma or nonseminoma.
- Computed tomography scans of the abdomen and pelvis are obtained to determine the presence of retroperitoneal lymphadenopathy, the initial route of spread of testicular germ cell tumors. Pathologic retroperitoneal lymphadenopathy is generally considered to be >1 cm in size. The site of lymph node metastases ("landing zones") can be predicted

based on the site of the primary tumor due to known venous drainage patterns:

- Left-sided tumors spread to the paraaortic lymph nodes, preaortic lymph nodes, and renal hilar lymph nodes.
- Right-sided tumors spread to the interaortocaval lymph nodes, precaval lymph nodes, and paraaortic lymph nodes.
- Chest imaging with a chest x-ray or computed tomography scan is obtained to evaluate for the presence of pulmonary metastases.

- Tumor markers
  - Three serum tumor markers have an established role in the diagnosis, prognostication, and monitoring of testicular germ cell tumors: alfa-fetoprotein (AFP), human chorionic gonadotropin (HCG), and lactate dehydrogenase (LDH).
  - AFP and/or β-HCG is elevated in approximately 85% of patients with nonseminomatous germ cell tumors.
  - β-HCG is elevated in less than 20% of patients with pure seminoma.
  - AFP is not elevated in patients with seminoma. Patients with a pathologic specimen interpreted as revealing a seminoma, but with an elevated AFP, should be treated for nonseminoma.

- Radical inguinal orchiectomy
  - A radical inguinal orchiectomy is the procedure of choice for the management of a suspected testicular germ cell tumor. This procedure is of both diagnostic and therapeutic value and may provide definitive management for patients with early-stage disease.
  - Transscrotal biopsies are not performed given concerns for tumor seeding and altered lymphatic drainage patterns.

■ Pathology of Testicular Carcinomas

- Germ cell tumors account for 95% of testicular tumors.
- The majority of germ cell tumors arise in the testes. However, germ cell tumors may also arise in the retro-

Table 13.1   Differences Between Seminomas and Nonseminomas

Seminoma
- Majority (≈85%) localized at presentation
- Sensitive to radiation
- Tumor markers typically not elevated (β-HCG is elevated in <20%; AFP is not elevated)

Nonseminoma
- Approximately 50% metastatic at presentation
- Resistant to radiation
- Commonly associated with elevated tumor markers

HCG, human chorionic gonadotropin; AFP, alfa-fetoprotein.

Table 13.2   Origin of Various Histologies of Germ Cell Tumors

Primordial Germ Cell					
Sperma-togonia	Seminoma	Embryonal carcinoma			
		Extraembryonic differentiation		Somatic differentiation	
		Chorio-carcinoma	Yolk sac tumor	Mature teratoma	Immature teratoma

peritoneum or mediastinum without evidence of a testicular primary. Many of these patients will have an occult or "burned out" testicular primary.

▪ Germ cell tumors are classified as seminomas or nonseminomas (see **Table 13.1**). The ratio of seminomas to nonseminomas is roughly 1:1. If there are any nonseminomatous elements present, the tumor is characterized and treated as a nonseminoma, regardless of the presence of seminomatous elements. Primordial germ cells can give rise to either seminoma or embryonal carcinoma (see **Table 13.2**). Embryonal carcinoma can differentiate into other histologies or teratoma.

- Seminomas
  - Account for approximately 50% of testicular germ cell tumors.
  - Tumor markers can be normal, or β-HCG may be elevated. If AFP is elevated, the tumor is characterized and treated as a nonseminoma (even if the pathology suggests a pure seminoma).
  - Anaplastic and spermatocytic seminomas are two histologic variants of seminoma.
- Nonseminomas
  - Approximately one-third of germ cell tumors are composed of combinations of the various histologic subtypes.
  - Embryonal carcinoma
  - Yolk sac tumor
    - Associated with elevated AFP
  - Choriocarcinoma
    - Associated with elevated β-HCG
  - Teratoma
    - Teratomas are tumors that have undergone differentiation to form somatic-type tissues typical of adult or fetal development.
    - There is little clinical utility to the distinction of mature and immature teratomas in testicular germ cell tumors.
    - Teratomas arise from malignant germ cell tumors and should be classified and treated as fully malignant nonseminomatous germ cell tumors, even if the cells of origin (e.g., embryonal carcinoma) are not detected in the pathology specimen.
    - Teratomatous elements can occasionally undergo malignant transformation (e.g., adenocarcinoma) and metastasize.
- Other (non–germ cell) testicular tumors
  - Sex cord stromal tumors
    - Account for <5% of testicular cancers in men
    - Leydig cell tumors
    - Sertoli cell tumors
    - Granulosa cell tumors

- Tumors of the paratesticular tissue
  - Mesothelioma
  - Lymphoma
    - Most common cause of a testicular mass in men older than 60 years.

Isochromosome 12p and Germ Cell Tumors

- An isochromosome of chromosome 12 is the most common and specific cytogenetic abnormality found in testicular germ cell tumors and is detectable in approximately 80% of patients.[1]
- Testing for isochromosome 12p should be considered for patients with poorly differentiated midline carcinomas of unknown primary site. The presence of isochromosome 12p in this setting is associated with a response to cisplatin-based therapy.[2]

Staging of Testicular Germ Cell Tumors (See Tables 13.3, 13.4, and 13.5.)

- The primary testicular tumor is staged surgically. The retroperitoneal lymph nodes may be staged either clinically (e.g., based on the results of a CT scan) or pathologically, depending on whether the patient has undergone a retroperitoneal lymph node dissection.
- The S stage (see Table 13.5) is based on the level of the tumor markers after orchiectomy. The S stage should not be assigned until the markers have been followed to determine if they are declining at their expected half-lives. For example, a β-HCG level of 400 on the day after an orchiectomy is performed does not necessarily indicate a stage of S1. The β-HCG should be followed with serial measurements. Based on the half-life of β-HCG, the value would be expected to normalize in approximately 8 days. If the value does not fall to normal, plateaus, or rises, the S stage is assigned. The half-lives of AFP and β-HCG are as follows:
  - AFP: approximately 5–7 days
  - HCG: approximately 30 hours

Table 13.3   TNM Staging in Testicular Germ Cell Cancer

T Stage (Primary Tumor)

pT1	Tumor limited to the testis and epididymis without vascular/lymphatic invasion; tumor may invade into the tunica albuginea but not the tunica vaginalis
pT2	Tumor limited to the testis and epididymis with vascular/lymphatic invasion, or tumor extending through the tunica albuginea with involvement of the tunica vaginalis
pT3	Tumor invades the spermatic cord with or without vascular/lymphatic invasion
pT4	Tumor invades the scrotum with or without vascular/lymphatic invasion

N Stage (Regional Lymph Nodes)

N0	No regional lymph node metastases are detected
N1	Metastasis with a lymph node mass 2 cm or less in greatest dimension; or multiple lymph nodes, none more than 2 cm in greatest dimension
N2	Metastasis with a lymph node mass more than 2 cm but not more than 5 cm in greatest dimension; or more than five nodes positive, none more than 5 cm; or evidence of extranodal extension of tumor
N3	Metastases with a lymph node mass more than 5 cm in greatest dimension

M Stage (Distant Metastasis)

M0	No distant metastasis
M1	Distant metastasis
	M1a—Nonregional nodal or pulmonary metastasis
	M1b—Distant metastasis other than to nonregional lymph nodes and lungs

Source: Used with the permission of the American Joint Committee on Cancer (AJCC), Chicago, Illinois. The original source for this material is the *AJCC Cancer Staging Manual,* Seventh Edition (2010), published by Springer Science and Business Media LLC, www.springer.com.

Table 13.4   Tumor Marker Staging in Testicular Cancer

	LDH	HCG	AFP
S1	<1.5 ULN	<5,000	<1,000
S2	1.5–10 × ULN	5,000–50,000	1,000–10,000
S3	>10 × ULN	>50,000	>10.000

LDH, lactate dehydrogenase; HCG, human chorionic gonadotropin; AFP, alfa-fetoprotein; ULN, upper limit of normal.

Source: Used with the permission of the American Joint Committee on Cancer (AJCC), Chicago, Illinois. The original source for this material is the *AJCC Cancer Staging Manual,* Sixth Edition (2002), published by Springer Science and Business Media LLC, www.springerlink.com.

Table 13.5   Testicular Germ Cell Cancer Stage Groupings

Stage Grouping	T Stage	N Stage	M Stage	S Stage
IA	pT1	N0	M0	S0
IB	pT2–4	N0	M0	S0
IS	Any T	N0	M0	S1–3
IIA	Any T	N1	M0	S0–1
IIB	Any T	N2	M0	S0–1
IIC	Any T	N3	M0	S0–1
IIIA	Any T	Any N	M1a	S0–1
IIIB	Any T	N1–3	M0	S2
	Any T	Any N	M1a	S2
IIIC	Any T	N1–3	M0	S3
	Any T	Any N	M1a	S3
	Any T	Any N	M1b	Any S

Source: Used with the permission of the American Joint Committee on Cancer (AJCC), Chicago, Illinois. The original source for this material is the *AJCC Cancer Staging Manual,* Seventh Edition (2010), published by Springer Science and Business Media LLC, www.springer.com.

■ References

1. Bosl GJ, Ilson DH, Rodriguez E, et al. Clinical relevance of the i(12p) marker chromosome in germ cell tumors. *J Natl Cancer Inst*. 1994;86:349–355.
2. Motzer RJ, Rodriguez E, Reuter VE, et al. Molecular and cytogenetic studies in the diagnosis of patients with poorly differentiated carcinomas of unknown primary site. *J Clin Oncol*. 1995;13:274–282.

Management of Stages I and II Seminoma

■ Stage I Seminoma

- Stage I seminomas are confined to the testis.
- There are three major management options for stage I seminomas: surveillance, radiation therapy, and chemotherapy.
  - Surveillance
    - Withholding adjuvant chemotherapy or radiation affords the opportunity to spare the potential morbidity of treatment for patients cured with surgery alone.
    - Approximately 15% of patients will relapse, the majority in the retroperitoneal lymph nodes.
    - Patients relapsing on surveillance can be effectively salvaged with radiation therapy or chemotherapy with no apparent detriment in outcomes compared with patients treated with adjuvant therapy.[1]
    - Success with a surveillance approach requires a motivated, compliant patient. A common surveillance strategy includes history and physical examination with serum tumor markers every 3–4 months for years 1–3, every 6 months for years 4–7, and then annually. Abdominal/pelvic CT scans are performed at each visit, with chest radiographs every other visit.
  - Radiation therapy
    - Historically, a "dog-leg" field was utilized to encompass the ipsilateral renal hilum, pelvic lymph nodes, and bilateral paraaortic nodes. This approach led to relapse rates of only 2–5%. The vast majority of relapsed patients were salvaged with chemotherapy,

resulting in a 10-year overall survival rate of 94–100%.[2] Long-term morbidity including impaired fertility and second malignancies led to studies exploring smaller radiation fields and lower doses.

- Given that the paraaortic lymph nodes are generally the first to be involved in patients with seminoma, limited radiation therapy to the paraaortic strip was explored. A randomized study comparing paraaortic radiation to dog-leg radiation demonstrated that paraaortic radiation was associated with reduced hematologic, gastrointestinal, and gonadal toxicity.[3] There was a higher risk of pelvic recurrence with paraaortic radiation, but no difference in overall survival between the groups. Paraaortic radiation has been accepted as a standard approach for patients with stage I seminoma pursuing adjuvant radiation.

- Radiation is typically administered in doses of 1.25–1.5 Gy per day to a total of 25–25.5 Gy.

- Although most men will return to baseline semen quality within approximately 2 years, cryopreservation of sperm should be offered prior to radiation therapy to allow assisted reproduction for patients who are infertile after radiation therapy.

- Men treated for seminoma have an increased risk of second malignancies, particularly solid tumors within the radiation field. The relative risk for men treated with adjuvant radiation therapy alone is 2.0.[4] The risk of second malignancies is likely less with newer radiation therapy techniques.

- The risk of cardiovascular disease is increased in men treated for seminoma, even in patients not receiving mediastinal radiation.

- Adjuvant chemotherapy
  - Several single-arm studies have explored one to two cycles of adjuvant carboplatin for treatment of stage I seminoma. Based on promising results, a phase III trial was conducted that randomized patients with stage I seminoma to adjuvant radiation therapy or a single dose of carboplatin (885 and 560 patients received radiotherapy and carboplatin, respectively).[5]

With a median follow-up of 4 years, relapse-free survival rates for radiotherapy and carboplatin were similar. There were no treatment-related deaths in either arm. There were significantly more second primary testicular tumors in patients treated with radiation.

- Retrospective analyses suggest a lower risk of relapse with two cycles of carboplatin compared with one cycle.

● Surveillance, radiation, and chemotherapy are all appropriate options for patients with clinical stage I seminoma after orchiectomy. The decision for treatment should be individualized based on the patient's ability to comply with a surveillance schedule and patient preferences regarding "active" treatment modalities.

■ Stage II Seminoma

- Men with stage II seminoma have radiographic involvement of the retroperitoneal lymph nodes. Treatment options depend somewhat on the bulk of retroperitoneal involvement, with N2 disease indicating lymph nodes of 2–5 cm in size and N3 disease indicating lymph nodes >5 cm in size.

- Stage IIA (N1) and IIB (N2)
  ● Radiation therapy to the paraaortic and ipsilateral iliac lymph nodes results in a disease-free survival rate of approximately 80–90% and a disease-specific survival rate of 90–100%. Approximately 40% of patients who relapse after receiving radiation therapy are effectively salvaged with chemotherapy.[6]
  ● Potential side effects of radiation therapy are as outlined in the section above on stage I seminoma.
  ● Some oncologists recommend chemotherapy, rather than radiation therapy, for patients with N2 disease. Chemotherapy with BEP (bleomycin, etoposide, and cisplatin) or EP (etoposide and cisplatin) has been explored in single-arm studies as an alternative to radiation therapy in patients with stage IIA and IIB disease, given concerns regarding long-term side effects

of radiation therapy. Preliminary results report a 4-year overall survival rate of 98% with this approach.

■ Stage IIC (N3) or Retroperitoneal Relapse After Radiation Therapy

- Chemotherapy is the mainstay of treatment for patients with stage IIC disease and for those patients who relapse after receiving adjuvant radiation therapy.
- Cisplatin-based combination chemotherapy with four cycles of EP or three cycles of BEP is standard treatment. The 3-year survival rate in stage IIC with these regimens is approximately 90%.
- The management of residual radiographic masses after chemotherapy is detailed below.

■ Stage III Seminoma

■ Men with stage III seminoma have metastases beyond the retroperitoneal lymph nodes.

■ Men with stage III seminoma are treated similarly to men with stage III nonseminoma (see Chapter 16).

■ Management of Postchemotherapy Residual Masses in Seminoma

■ Residual radiographic abnormalities postchemotherapy are encountered in up to 80% of men treated for seminoma.

■ Traditionally, the size of the residual mass was utilized as a predictor of the presence of viable tumor and the need for additional therapy.

■ Prospective data support the use of fluorodeoxyglucose positron emission tomography (FDG-PET) scanning for evaluation of postchemotherapy residual masses in seminoma.[7] The SEMPET study explored PET scans in 51 patients with residual radiographic abnormalities on CT scan after chemotherapy for seminoma. The PET scan results were correlated with either histology at the time of resection of the residual mass or outcome based on clinical follow-up. All 19 cases with residual lesions >3 cm and 35 of 37 with residual lesions >3 cm were correctly predicted by PET. The specificity, sensitivity, positive predictive value, and negative predictive value of FDG-PET were 100%, 80%, 100%, and 96%, respectively. Based on these data, patients with FDG-avid residual disease on PET scan are generally managed with additional treatment (e.g., surgery or radiation therapy), whereas those patients without FDG-avid masses are observed.

- The utility of PET scanning for evaluation of posttreatment residual masses in nonseminoma has been less impressive because teratoma remains in the differential diagnosis of a residual mass in patients with nonseminoma, and teratoma is generally not FDG-avid.

■ References

1. Choo R, Thomas G, Woo T, et al. Long-term outcome of postorchiectomy surveillance for stage I testicular seminoma. *Int J Radiat Oncol Biol Phys.* 2005;61:736–740.
2. Dosmann MA, Zagars GK. Post-orchiectomy radiotherapy for stages I and II testicular seminoma. *Int J Radiat Oncol Biol Phys.* 1993;26:381–390.
3. Fossa SD, Horwich A, Russell JM, et al. Optimal planning target volume for stage I testicular seminoma: a Medical Research Council randomized trial. Medical Research Council Testicular Tumor Working Group. *J Clin Oncol.* 1999;17:1146.
4. Travis LB, Curtis RE, Storm H, et al. Risk of second malignant neoplasms among long-term survivors of testicular cancer. *J Natl Cancer Inst.* 1997;89:1429–1439.
5. Oliver RT, Mason MD, Mead GM, et al. Radiotherapy versus single-dose carboplatin in adjuvant treatment of stage I seminoma: a randomised trial. *Lancet.* 2005;366:293–300.
6. Whipple GL, Sagerman RH, van Rooy EM. Long-term evaluation of postorchiectomy radiotherapy for stage II seminoma. *Am J Clin Oncol.* 1997;20:196–201.
7. De Santis M, Becherer A, Bokemeyer C, et al. 2-18fluoro-deoxy-D-glucose positron emission tomography is a reliable predictor for viable tumor in postchemotherapy seminoma: an update of the prospective multicentric SEMPET trial. *J Clin Oncol.* 2004;22:1034–1039.

Management of Stages I and II Nonseminoma

■ Clinical Stage I Nonseminoma

- Stage I nonseminomas are confined to the testis. The serum tumor markers must be within normal limits or, if initially elevated, must have returned to normal with serial measurements after orchiectomy. If the serum tumor markers are persistently elevated (not declining at the expected half-life) or are rising after orchiectomy, the patient should be treated for stage IS disease.

- There are three major management options for stage I nonseminomas: surveillance, retroperitoneal lymph node dissection (RPLND), and adjuvant chemotherapy. Given the ability to successfully employ salvage treatment for patients who develop recurrent disease, there are no clear differences in survival with each of these approaches, and cure rates are approximately 98%. The appropriate option for an individual patient depends on the presence of risk factors for micrometastatic disease to the retroperitoneal lymph nodes, ability to comply with a strict surveillance strategy, availability of a urologist with substantial experience in performing retroperitoneal lymph node dissections, and patient preference.

  - Surveillance
    - Approximately 20–25% of men undergoing surveillance after orchiectomy for a nonseminomatous germ cell tumor will develop a relapse. The vast majority of these patients (≈95%) will be effectively salvaged, most commonly with chemotherapy.
    - Pathologic risk factors are somewhat helpful in determining which patients are at highest risk of micrometastatic disease to the retroperitoneal

lymph nodes. In an analysis of 200 patients with clinical stage I seminoma prospectively assigned to RPLND, the presence of vascular invasion was the most predictive of pathologic stage II disease on multivariate analysis.[1] However, the positive predictive value was only 52%. Therefore, even in men with "high risk" clinical stage I disease, a large proportion will be overtreated with RPLND. Other commonly utilized risk factors for relapse include pT2–3 disease or a large component of embryonal carcinoma in the primary tumor. There are institutional variations in the use of these risk factors as criteria for recommending treatment versus surveillance. Many centers continue to recommend treatment (primarily RPLND, although some oncologists recommend chemotherapy, see below) for patients with any of the following risk factors: vascular invasion, predominant component of embryonal carcinoma, or pT2–3 disease.

- For surveillance to be successful (without compromising curability), patients must be compliant and adhere to a strict schedule of follow-up visits and radiographic evaluations. A common surveillance strategy includes history and physical examinations, chest radiographs, and serum tumor marker levels every other month for the first 2 years, every 4 months in the third year, every 6 months in the fourth year, and then annually. Abdominal CT scans are performed every 4 months for the first 2 years, then every 6–12 months.
- Studies have suggested compliance rates with surveillance as low as 35%.[2]
- RPLND
  - Surgical dissection of the retroperitoneal lymph nodes represents an effective treatment option given the predictable pattern of spread of germ cell tumors.
  - Given the risk for retrograde ejaculation with older techniques, a nerve-sparing RPLND is now

commonly employed. With this technique, the nerves responsible for ejaculation are spared, with the goal of preserving fertility.

▪ For men with pathologic evidence of extensive micrometastases, adjuvant chemotherapy should be considered (see stage II disease below).

▪ The risk of recurrence for men with stage I non-seminoma germ cell tumor (NSGCT) post-RPLND is approximately 5%. The vast majority of these relapses occur outside of the retroperitoneum. Therefore, surveillance post-RPLND is still required, albeit with a less-intensive schedule than for patients seeking primary surveillance. A common surveillance strategy involves a physical exam, chest x-ray, and tumor markers every 3 months for the first year, every 6 months for the second year, and then annually. A CT scan of the abdomen and pelvis is obtained annually for 3 years.

• Chemotherapy

▪ Chemotherapy with one or two cycles of BEP is an alternative treatment approach for patients with "high risk" clinical stage I NSGCT.

▪ Potential advantages of chemotherapy for clinical stage I NSGCT:

• Most oncologists have extensive experience with the administration of these chemotherapeutic agents; as a result, the treatment is widely available. This is in contrast to an RPLND, which is more commonly performed at referral centers.

• Patients who relapse after RPLND generally require treatment with a full course of chemotherapy (three to four cycles) rather than the one to two cycles that are administered as "adjuvant" chemotherapy.

▪ Potential disadvantages of chemotherapy for clinical stage I NSGCT:

• The acute and chronic toxicities of chemotherapy may be lessened with an abbreviated course of one to two cycles. However, mild hearing loss, decrease in pulmonary diffusion capacity, and peripheral neuropathy have been reported following two cycles of BEP. Furthermore, several studies exploring chemotherapy for clinical stage I NSGCT have had insufficient follow-up, and potential late toxicities are of concern.

- Chemotherapy does not effectively treat teratoma. As a result, teratoma in the retroperitoneum may progress slowly over time, with the potential for malignant transformation. Despite this concern, an increase in late relapses/malignant transformation has not been reported in chemotherapy series thus far.

- The German Multicenter Prospective Trial randomized 382 patients to either one cycle of BEP or RPLND.[3] Patients undergoing RPLND with evidence of pathologic retroperitoneal lymph node involvement (pathologic stage II) received two cycles of postoperative BEP. After a median follow-up of 4.7 years, 2 and 15 recurrences were observed in the intention-to-treat population with chemotherapy and surgery, respectively ($p = 0.0011$). The difference in the 2-year recurrence-free survival rate between chemotherapy (99.46%; 95% CI 96.20–99.92%) and surgery (91.87%; 95% CI 86.87–95.02%) was 7.59% (95% CI 3.13–12.05%). The hazard ratio to experience a tumor recurrence with surgery as opposed to chemotherapy was 7.937 (95% CI 1.808–34.48). There was no difference in disease-specific or overall survival. Which strategy results in the best long-term outcomes, with the least late complications, is not clear given the short follow-up available from this study.

- Several single-arm studies have evaluated two cycles of BEP as adjuvant therapy. The optimal number of cycles of chemotherapy in patients with clinical stage I NSGCT remains unclear.

■ Clinical Stage IS Nonseminoma

▪ Patients with elevated or rising tumor markers after orchiectomy (and a period of observation to determine if the markers are declining at the expected half-life to the normal range) should be treated for metastatic disease with chemotherapy despite the absence of radiographic metastases on imaging.

▪ Patients with stage IS NSGCT should be treated with three cycles of BEP or four cycles of EP.

■ Clinical Stage II Nonseminoma

▪ Patients with clinical stage II NSGCT have radiographic evidence of retroperitoneal lymphadenopathy.

▪ Patients with clinical stage II NSGCT and elevated tumor markers should be treated with chemotherapy according to risk stratification (see Chapter 16).

▪ For patients with clinical stage II NSGCT and normal tumor markers, both RPLND and chemotherapy are acceptable approaches, with many centers using different criteria for which patients are best treated with each modality. Retroperitoneal lymph node dissection is often favored in patients with clinical stage IIA NSGCT because a significant proportion of these patients will not have evidence of pathologic involvement of the retroperitoneal lymph nodes (pathologic stage I disease). On the other hand, although RPLND is curative in 80–90% of patients with clinical stage IIA NSGCT, approximately 65% of patients with clinical stage IIB–C disease are cured. Therefore, many centers advocate primary chemotherapy for patients with stage IIB–C disease (with four cycles of EP or three cycles of BEP).

  • Risk stratification has also been utilized to determine which patients should be treated with RPLND versus primary chemotherapy. One approach has been to recommend chemotherapy in patients with retroperitoneal lymphadenopathy larger than 2 cm, multiple masses, or disease outside the primary landing zone.[4]

- Patients treated with RPLND with evidence of extensive pathologic involvement should receive post-RPLND chemotherapy (see "Pathologic Stage II Nonseminoma").
- Patients treated with primary chemotherapy should undergo postchemotherapy RPLND to resect any residual radiographic disease (with some centers advocating RPLND in all patients with postchemotherapy). The etiology of postchemotherapy residual masses includes:
  - Fibrosis: approximately 50%
  - Teratoma: approximately 30–40%
  - Viable tumor: approximately 10–20%

■ Pathologic Stage II Nonseminoma

- Patients with pathologic stage II NSGCT have evidence of pathologic involvement of the retroperitoneal lymph nodes.
- Adjuvant chemotherapy post-RPLND or surveillance are acceptable approaches for patients with pathologic stage II NSGCT.
- A randomized multinational study compared immediate adjuvant chemotherapy versus chemotherapy at the time of relapse in patients with pathologic stage II NSGCT.[5] There were more frequent relapses in patients on the surveillance arm (48 of 98 versus 6 of 97), but no difference in survival because patients relapsing on surveillance were effectively salvaged with chemotherapy.
- Patients with higher-volume pathologic lymph node involvement are at higher risk for relapse. As a result, surveillance is commonly employed for patients with pathologic stage IIA disease, whereas two cycles of adjuvant EP or BEP are recommended for patients with pathologic stage IIB or IIC disease.

■ Stage III Nonseminoma

- Men with stage III nonseminoma have metastases beyond the retroperitoneal lymph nodes.
- See Chapter 16 for more information about treatment of stage III nonseminoma.

■ References

1. Albers P, Siener R, Kliesch S, et al. Risk factors for relapse in clinical stage I nonseminomatous testicular germ cell tumors: results of the German Testicular Cancer Study Group Trial. *J Clin Oncol.* 2003;21:1505–1512.
2. Hao D, Seidel J, Brant R, et al. Compliance of clinical stage I nonseminomatous germ cell tumor patients with surveillance. *J Urol.* 1998;160:768–771.
3. Albers P, Siener R, Krege S, et al. Randomized phase III trial comparing retroperitoneal lymph node dissection with one course of bleomycin and etoposide plus cisplatin chemotherapy in the adjuvant treatment of clinical stage I nonseminomatous testicular germ cell tumors: AUO trial AH 01/94 by the German Testicular Cancer Study Group. *J Clin Oncol.* 2008;26:2966–2972.
4. Stephenson AJ, Bosl GJ, Motzer RJ, et al. Nonrandomized comparison of primary chemotherapy and retroperitoneal lymph node dissection for clinical stage IIA and IIB nonseminomatous germ cell testicular cancer. *J Clin Oncol.* 2007;25:5597–5602.
5. Williams SD, Stablein DM, Einhorn LH, et al. Immediate adjuvant chemotherapy versus observation with treatment at relapse in pathological stage II testicular cancer. *N Engl J Med.* 1987;317:1433–1438.

Management of Advanced and Recurrent Germ Cell Tumors

■ Stage III Seminoma and Nonseminoma

- Men with stage III seminoma and nonseminoma have metastases beyond the retroperitoneal lymph nodes and are potentially curable with chemotherapy with or without surgical resection of residual disease.

- Treatment with BEP for four cycles became the standard regimen for metastatic germ cell tumors after a randomized trial compared this regimen with the prior standard, PVB (cisplatin, vinblastine, bleomycin).[1] In this trial, BEP was associated with less neuromuscular toxicity and a higher complete response rate in patients with "high volume" disease.

- Given the high rate of curability with advanced germ cell tumors, much effort over the past two decades has focused on risk-stratifying patients to determine which patients may be cured with less-intense therapy (thereby minimizing potential short- and long-term toxicity) and which patients may need more aggressive treatment to achieve cure. An international effort led to a validated prognostic model for patients with advanced germ cell tumors (see **Table 16.1**).[2] This model assigns patients with advanced seminoma into good or intermediate risk categories and patients with nonseminoma into good-, intermediate-, or poor-risk categories. These categories not only are of prognostic significance, but also are important in treatment selection.

Table 16.1 Risk Stratification in Advanced Germ Cell Tumors

	Good Risk	Intermediate Risk	Poor Risk
Nonseminoma	■ Testicular or RP primary ■ No nonpulmonary visceral metastases ■ AFP <1,000 ■ HCG <5,000 ■ LDH <1.53 ULN	■ Testicular or RP primary ■ No nonpulmonary visceral metastases ■ AFP 1,000–10,000 ■ HCG 5,000–50,000 ■ LDH 1.5–10 × ULN	■ Mediastinal primary ■ Nonpulmonary visceral metastases ■ AFP > 10,000 ■ HCG > 50,000 ■ LDH > 10 × ULN
Seminoma	■ Any primary site ■ No nonpulmonary visceral metastases ■ Normal AFP; any LDH or HCG	■ Any primary site ■ Nonpulmonary visceral metastases ■ Normal AFP; any LDH or HCG	No poor-risk seminoma subgroup
5-year survival	91%	79%	48%

RP, retroperitoneal; AFP, alfa-fetoprotein; HCG, human chorionic gonadotropin; LDH, lactate dehydrogenase; ULN, upper limit of normal.

Source: Data derived from International Germ Cell Cancer Collaborative Group.[2]

- Good-risk disease
  - Approximately 90% of patients with good-risk germ cell tumors are cured with chemotherapy (with or without surgical resection of residual disease).
  - Several randomized trials have explored modified chemotherapy regimens in an attempt to reduce the potential toxicity of treatment for patients with good-risk disease (see **Table 16.2**). Only the reduction in the number of cycles of BEP (from four cycles to three) has been widely adopted as standard therapy for this subgroup of patient. The use of four cycles of EP remains controversial but is advocated at Memorial Sloan-Kettering Cancer Center based on randomized data demonstrating no statistically significant detriment in survival and a reduced risk of Raynaud phenomenon, cardiovascular toxicity, and pulmonary toxicity.[6,7]
- Intermediate-risk and poor-risk disease
  - BEP for four cycles is standard treatment for patients with intermediate-risk and poor-risk germ cell tumors.
  - Several approaches have been explored in an attempt to improve outcomes in patients with intermediate- or poor-risk disease.

Table 16.2   Selected Randomized Trials in Patients with Good-Risk Germ Cell Tumors

Treatment Arms	Conclusions
BEP × 3 cycles vs. BEP × 3 cycles[6]	BEP × 3 was associated with less toxicity and similar efficacy to BEP × 4.
BEP × 4 cycles vs. EP × 4 cycles[4]	Higher mortality on the EP × 4 arm did not reach statistical significance (trial underpowered for survival).
BEP × 4 cycles vs. BEC × 4 cycles[7]	The carboplatin arm was inferior to the cisplatin arm.

BEP, bleomycin, etoposide, cisplatin; BEC, bleomycin, etoposide, carboplatin; EP, etoposide plus cisplatin.

- Given the efficacy of VIP (etoposide, ifosfamide, cisplatin) in patients with relapsed disease, a randomized trial compared four cycles of VIP with four cycles of BEP as first-line treatment in patients with intermediate- and poor-risk germ cell tumors.[8] There was no difference in outcomes between the two arms, and toxicity was slightly worse with VIP.
- High-dose chemotherapy with autologous stem cell transplantation has also been demonstrated to cure a proportion of patients with relapsed germ cell tumors. As a result, a randomized trial compared four cycles of BEP with two cycles of BEP followed by high-dose chemotherapy and autologous stem cell transplantation as first-line treatment in patients with intermediate- and poor-risk germ cell tumors.[9] The 1-year complete response rate was 52% for the high-dose therapy arm and 48% for the BEP-alone arm ($p = 0.53$).

■ Postchemotherapy Resection of Residual Disease

- With rare exception, postchemotherapy surgery in patients with germ cell tumors should only be performed in patients with normalized tumor markers. Patients with elevated or rising tumor markers require additional chemotherapy.
- The management of postchemotherapy residual radiographic masses in the retroperitoneum in patients with stage II seminoma and nonseminoma is discussed in Chapters 14 and 15, respectively.
- In patients with advanced germ cell tumors and normalized tumor markers after chemotherapy, all residual disease should be resected if feasible. Residual masses are most commonly teratoma or fibrosis, although viable tumor may also be found. Teratoma is not chemosensitive and has the potential to undergo malignant transformation, underscoring the importance of resecting residual masses.

▓ Side Effects of Chemotherapy for Germ Cell Tumors

▓ Bleomycin pulmonary toxicity
  • Pulmonary toxicity from bleomycin accounts for approximately half of treatment-related deaths in men with germ cell tumors treated with chemotherapy.
  • The incidence of fatal pulmonary toxicity from bleomycin is <1% with three cycles of BEP and 1–2% with four cycles of BEP.
  • Pulmonary function tests (with diffusion capacity) are obtained prior to initiating treatment with bleomycin. Most oncologists recommend discontinuing bleomycin if the diffusion capacity decreases by 40% during the course of therapy.
  • Bleomycin lung toxicity may manifest as the development of pulmonary nodules. Therefore, pulmonary nodules that develop during the course of therapy should be evaluated carefully and not assumed to be related to malignancy.
▓ Renal impairment
  • Acute and chronic renal impairment are potential side effects of treatment with cisplatin. In a study of late toxicity of germ cell tumor treatment, an average decline in creatinine clearance of approximately 15% was observed.[10]
▓ Ototoxicity
  • Hearing loss and tinnitus are potential side effects of treatment with cisplatin. In a study of late toxicity of germ cell tumor treatment, there was considerable effect on long-term audiometric function, but frequencies affected were outside the range of conversational speech.[10]
▓ Alopecia
  • Alopecia develops in virtually all patients treated with chemotherapy for germ cell tumors and is reversible.
▓ Infertility
  • Many men with germ cell tumors have impaired fertility at baseline, which may be further compounded by orchiectomy.

- Chemotherapy for germ cell tumors is associated with a dose-dependent impairment in spermatogenesis.
- In a study of men receiving chemotherapy for germ cell tumors, the likelihood of achieving normal sperm counts (in patients with normal baseline sperm counts) was 22% and 58% at 2 and 5 years from treatment, respectively.[11]
- Sperm banking is recommended in patients with germ cell tumors prior to initiating chemotherapy.
- Vascular toxicity
  - Men treated with chemotherapy for germ cell tumors are at increased risk for several vascular toxicities, including:
    - Hypertension
    - Hyperlipidemia
    - Coronary artery disease
    - Raynaud phenomenon
    - Thromboembolic disease

Relapsed and Refractory Germ Cell Tumors

- The majority of men with relapsed germ cell tumors are initially diagnosed due to rising tumor markers.
- In men undergoing surveillance for stage I seminoma or nonseminoma, salvage treatment depends on the extent and location of disease. Patients relapsing with seminoma or nonseminoma in the retroperitoneum are treated as outlined for patients with stage II disease in Chapters 14 and 15.
- For men relapsing after prior chemotherapy, several regimens have been explored. The choice of regimen and the timing of high-dose chemotherapy and stem cell transplant are controversial. Prognostic factors may be helpful in determining which patients may be best treated with standard-dose salvage chemotherapy and which patients are better treated with high-dose chemotherapy and autologous stem cell transplantation at first relapse. For example, a testicular primary tumor and a prior complete response to first-line chemotherapy have been identified as favorable prognostic factors for standard-dose salvage therapy.

- Standard-dose chemotherapy
  - Ifosfamide-based regimens are most commonly employed for men with recurrent germ cell tumors after prior chemotherapy. Two main ifosfamide-based regimens have been explored: VeIP (vinblastine, ifosfamide, and cisplatin) and TIP (paclitaxel, ifosfamide, and cisplatin).
  - The activity of four cycles of TIP was explored in a phase II trial of 46 patients with progressive metastatic germ cell tumors.[12] Eligibility required that patients have a testicular primary tumor and had achieved a complete response to first-line chemotherapy. The 2-year progression-free survival rate was 65% (95% CI 51–79%).
- High-dose chemotherapy with autologous stem cell transplant
  - Single-center trials have explored various high-dose chemotherapy regimens as treatment for relapsed germ cell tumors.
    - A prospective study evaluated two cycles of ifosfamide plus paclitaxel followed by three cycles of high-dose carboplatin and etoposide (each supported by an autologous stem cell transplant).[13] All patients had unfavorable prognostic factors for achieving a complete response to standard-dose salvage therapy, including extragonadal primary site, progressive disease after an incomplete response to first-line therapy, and/or poor response or lack of response to prior treatment with cisplatin plus ifosfamide conventional-dose therapy. Twenty-nine (55%) of 47 patients achieved a complete response to chemotherapy with or without resection of residual disease; 24 patients (51%) were alive and free of disease at a median follow-up time of 40 months.
    - A retrospective study reported the Indiana University experience with high-dose carboplatin and etoposide and tandem autologous stem cell transplantation as salvage treatment for

relapsed germ cell tumors.14 At a median follow-up of 48 months, 94 of 135 patients who
received the treatment as second-line therapy
were disease-free, and 22 of 49 patients who
received treatment as third-line or later therapy
were disease-free.

■ In a randomized study, 280 patients were assigned to receive either four cycles of cisplatin, ifosfamide, and etoposide (or vinblastine)
or three cycles of this regimen followed by
one cycle of high-dose carboplatin, etoposide,
and cyclophosphamide and autologous stem
cell transplantation.[15] There was no difference in survival with the high-dose chemotherapy arm; however, the applicability of these
results to contemporary high-dose regimens is unclear because current regimens generally employ
two or three cycles of high-dose chemotherapy,
each supported with stem cell transplantation.

• Men who are refractory to initial chemotherapy, who
relapse within 4 weeks of completing initial cisplatin-
based chemotherapy, or who relapse after high-dose
chemotherapy have a very poor prognosis. However,
durable complete responses have been achieved in a
proportion of men with various regimens, including
gemcitabine plus paclitaxel, gemcitabine plus oxali-
platin, and epirubicin plus cisplatin.

■ Late relapses of germ cell tumors (relapses occurring
>2 years after completion of initial chemotherapy) have
been associated with a poor prognosis. Several reports
have suggested that the majority of late relapses occur
after 5 years. In a population-based study, relapses >5 years
from initial treatment occurred in 1.8% of men with nonseminoma and 0.8% of men with seminoma.[16] Although
late relapses are relatively uncommon, long-term survival
can be achieved in a proportion of patients treated with
chemotherapy and aggressive surgical resection, high-
lighting the need for ongoing surveillance for men treated
for germ cell tumors.

■ References

1. Williams SD, Birch R, Einhorn LH, et al. Treatment of disseminated germ-cell tumors with cisplatin, bleomycin, and either vinblastine or etoposide. *N Engl J Med*. 1987; 316:1435–1440.

2. International Germ Cell Cancer Collaborative Group. International Germ Cell Consensus Classification: a prognostic factor-based staging system for metastatic germ cell cancers. *J Clin Oncol*. 1997;15:594–603.

3. Einhorn LH, Williams SD, Loehrer PJ, et al. Evaluation of optimal duration of chemotherapy in favorable-prognosis disseminated germ cell tumors: a Southeastern Cancer Study Group protocol. *J Clin Oncol*. 1989;7:387–391.

4. Culine S, Kerbrat P, Kramar A, et al. Refining the optimal chemotherapy regimen for good-risk metastatic nonseminomatous germ-cell tumors: a randomized trial of the Genito-Urinary Group of the French Federation of Cancer Centers (GETUG T93BP). *Ann Oncol*. 2007;18:917–924.

5. Horwich A, Sleijfer DT, Fossa SD, et al. Randomized trial of bleomycin, etoposide, and cisplatin compared with bleomycin, etoposide, and carboplatin in good-prognosis metastatic nonseminomatous germ cell cancer: a multi-institutional Medical Research Council/European Organization for Research and Treatment of Cancer Trial. *J Clin Oncol*. 1997; 15:1844–1852.

6. Bosl GJ, Geller NL, Bajorin D, et al. A randomized trial of etoposide + cisplatin versus vinblastine + bleomycin + cisplatin + cyclophosphamide + dactinomycin in patients with good-prognosis germ cell tumors. *J Clin Oncol*. 1988; 6:1231–1238.

7. Kondagunta GV, Bacik J, Bajorin D, et al. Etoposide and cisplatin chemotherapy for metastatic good-risk germ cell tumors. *J Clin Oncol*. 2005;23:9290–9294.

8. Nichols CR, Catalano PJ, Crawford ED, et al. Randomized comparison of cisplatin and etoposide and either bleomycin or ifosfamide in treatment of advanced disseminated germ cell tumors: an Eastern Cooperative Oncology Group, Southwest Oncology Group, and Cancer and Leukemia Group B Study. *J Clin Oncol*. 1998;16:1287–1293.

9. Motzer RJ, Nichols CJ, Margolin KA, et al. Phase III randomized trial of conventional-dose chemotherapy with or without high-dose chemotherapy and autologous hematopoietic stem-cell rescue as first-line treatment for patients with poor-prognosis metastatic germ cell tumors. *J Clin Oncol*. 2007;25:247–256.

10. Osanto S, Bukman A, Van Hoek F, et al. Long-term effects of chemotherapy in patients with testicular cancer. *J Clin Oncol*. 1992;10:574–579.
11. Lampe H, Horwich A, Norman A, et al. Fertility after chemotherapy for testicular germ cell cancers. *J Clin Oncol*. 1997; 15:239–245.
12. Kondagunta GV, Bacik J, Donadio A, et al. Combination of paclitaxel, ifosfamide, and cisplatin is an effective second-line therapy for patients with relapsed testicular germ cell tumors. *J Clin Oncol*. 2005;23:6549–6555.
13. Kondagunta GV, Bacik J, Sheinfeld J, et al. Paclitaxel plus ifosfamide followed by high-dose carboplatin plus etoposide in previously treated germ cell tumors. *J Clin Oncol*. 2007; 25:85–90.
14. Einhorn LH, Williams SD, Chamness A, et al. High-dose chemotherapy and stem-cell rescue for metastatic germ-cell tumors. *N Engl J Med*. 2007;357:340–348.
15. Pico JL, Rosti G, Kramar A, et al. A randomised trial of high-dose chemotherapy in the salvage treatment of patients failing first-line platinum chemotherapy for advanced germ cell tumours. *Ann Oncol*. 2005;16:1152–1159.
16. Oldenburg J, Alfsen GC, Waehre H, et al. Late recurrences of germ cell malignancies: a population-based experience over three decades. *Br J Cancer*. 2006;94:820–827.

Common Treatment Regimens in Genitourinary Oncology

■ Urothelial Carcinoma

Gemcitabine + Cisplatin

Gemcitabine 1,000 mg/m^2 IV days 1, 8, and 15

Cisplatin 70 mg/m^2 IV day 1

Repeat cycle every 28 days (note: in clinical practice the day 15 dose of gemcitabine is often omitted and treatment is recycled every 21 days)

MVAC

Methotrexate 30 mg/m^2 IV days 1, 15, and 22

Vinblastine 3 mg/m^2 IV days 2, 15, and 22

Doxorubicin 30 mg/m^2 IV day 2

Cisplatin 70 mg/m^2 IV day 2

Repeat cycle every 28 days.

■ Renal Carcinoma

Sorafenib 400 mg orally twice daily

Sunitinib 50 mg orally daily for 4 weeks followed by 2 weeks rest

Pazopanib 800 mg orally daily

Temsirolimus 25 mg IV weekly

Everolimus 10 mg orally daily

■ Germ Cell Carcinoma

BEP

Bleomycin 30 units IV days 2, 9, and 16
Etoposide 100 mg/m^2 IV days 1–5
Cisplatin 20 mg/m^2 IV days 1–5
Repeat cycle every 21 days.

EP

Etoposide 100 mg/m^2 IV days 1–5
Cisplatin 20 mg/m^2 IV days 1–5
Repeat cycle every 21 days.

VeIP

Vinblastine 0.11 mg/kg IV days 1–2
Ifosfamide 1.2 g/m^2 IV days 1–5
Cisplatin 20 mg/m^2 IV days 1–5
Mesna
Repeat cycle every 21 days.

TIP

Paclitaxel 250 mg/m^2 IV day 1
Ifosfamide 1.5 g/m^2 IV days 2–5
Cisplatin 25 mg/m^2 IV days 2–5
Mesna
Filgrastim
Repeat cycle every 21 days.

Index